Low Back Disorders
A Medical Enigma

5

Low Back Disorders
A Medical Enigma

Rene Cailliet, M.D.
Professor Emeritus
University of Southern California
Keck School of Medicine;
Clinical Professor
School of Medicine
University of California at Los Angeles
Los Angeles, California

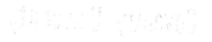
LIPPINCOTT WILLIAMS & WILKINS
A **Wolters Kluwer** Company
Philadelphia · Baltimore · New York · London
Buenos Aires · Hong Kong · Sydney · Tokyo

Acquisitions Editor: Robert Hurley
Developmental Editor: Joanne Bersin
Production Editor: Melanie Bennitt
Manufacturing Manager: Colin J. Warnock
Cover Designer: Joseph Piliero
Compositor: Circle Graphics
Printer: R. R. Donnelley–Crawfordsville

© **2003 by LIPPINCOTT WILLIAMS & WILKINS**
530 Walnut Street
Philadelphia, PA 19106 USA
LWW.com

Printed in the USA

Library of Congress Cataloging-in-Publication Data

Cailliet, Rene.
    Low back disorders : a medical enigma / Rene Cailliet.
        p. ; cm.
    Includes bibliographical references and index.
    ISBN 0-7817-4448-2
    1. Backache. 2. Backache—Pathophysiology. I. Title.
    [DNLM: 1. Low Back Pain—physiopathology. WE 755 C134La 2003]
    RD771.B217 .C347 2003
    617.5′6407—dc21

10 9 8 7 6 5 4 3 2 1

CONTENTS

PREFACE

At an international Forum for Primary Care Research on Low Back Pain in Israel (2000) (1) the comment was made that "researchers are on the verge of solving the back pain problem," but not all were in agreement.

Gordon Waddell, a Scottish orthopedic surgeon, stated, "Don't turn a subjective health complaint into a medical condition" (2). He implied that current medical thinking considers low back disability as a "disease," which it is not in the accepted sense of the word.

Peter Croft (2) from Britain noted, "There is scant evidence that any form of medical treatment can alter the natural history of the prevalent condition over the long term." It is the opinion of this author that there is management that can alter the "condition" if that condition were better understood.

In that same publication (2) Jeffrey Borkan, M.D., the chairperson, stated, "The traditional biomedical model of low back pain has generally proven to be a failure in primary care settings." A biomedical model should be replaced by a model with "impairment," not pain, as the primary goal of any intervention.

A "biopsychosocial" approach to low back disorders is gaining prevalence in the management of low back disorders. The "psychosocial" aspect of this approach gets precedence and the "bio" aspect is neglected. Both are pertinent. The psychosocial aspect affects the "bio" but the "bio" aspect needs clarification.

"Bio" must be understood to be the physical (mechanical) cause of dysfunction. Waddell aptly states that low back problems "may not be gross anatomic disruptions but rather are a disruption of neuromuscular function and neurophysiology." This disruption is an example of how the psychosocial intervenes upon the physiologic and is a disruption of neuromuscular function and neurophysiology. Unfortunately, the reasons remain unclear.

Voluminous literature on the problems of the low back has been written in recent decades with impairment primarily related to the disc of the spine and thus all studies and treatment protocols have been so directed. Management for the "condition" has involved numerous modalities and even surgical intervention. However, the results have been disappointing.

In an effort to review all the related international publications, the Cochrane Collaboration Back Review Group for Spinal Disorders was created in England in 1992 (3). This group publishes its results to answer the following questions: What works and what does not work in the treatment of back pain? What is the evidence and how strong is that evidence? How can a busy clinician distill this evidence and sort out the good? Subgroups of the Cochrane Collaboration Group remain active in many countries periodically reviewing all pertinent literature (1). All these studies pertain to the modification of the incurred pain and its disability, but little attention is given toward understanding how the low back normally functions and how malfunction can be evaluated and altered.

It is evident from review of this excessive literature that the low back remains a medical "enigma," without specific answers as to the cause, the value of elaborate examinations, or the effectiveness of numerous, prolonged, and expensive treatments. The magnitude of medical costs, personal injury claims, and industrial losses from this impairment is evidence that the problem remains unanswered. This text is offered as a possible answer to some of these questions.

The clinical biomechanics of the spine have been well documented and research concludes that the impairment leading to the claimed disability is from impaired biomechanics. Of the tissue or tissues that are allegedly damaged and causing impairment, attention is directed to the intervertebral disc and its related tissues, but the specific relationship between the damage and the symptoms remains unclear.

The discussion of a different concept of cause and effect is the culmination of 40 years of clinical practice and 30 years of writing. Many if not most of these proposed mechanisms are under the control of the person who becomes "injured." With a clearer understanding of the proposed mechanisms, the therapist and the patient will benefit from implementation of the proposed treatment protocols. Relief of the symptoms of the current episode of low back pain will be afforded and, more important, recurrence of another episode, which adversely influences a person's quality of life performance, can be prevented. Chronic pain, often without a recognized pathological basis, can be avoided.

A better understanding of these proposed mechanisms is aided by informative illustrations of the tissues and mechanisms that clarify this medical dilemma that has confused the public for so many centuries. The illustrations, all drawn by the author, are intentionally simplified to make the reader aware of the "functional" part of the spine that leads to disability often with pain.

Rene Cailliet, M.D.

REFERENCES

1. Cherkin DC, *et al*. A randomized trial comparing acupuncture, therapeutic massage and self-care education for chronic low back pain. Presented

at the Fourth International Forum for Primary Care Research on Low Back Pain. Eilat, Israel, 2000 (not yet published).
2. Waddell G, Burton AK. Occupational Health Guidelines for Management of Low Back Pain at Work-Evidence Review. London: Faculty of Occupational Medicine, 2000.
3. *The Back Letter*. Philadelphia: Lippincott Williams & Wilkins, 2000; 15:No.S.

FOREWORD

For recent decades, numerous opinions have arisen regarding the causation of low back disorders and even concentrated on the value of the numerous remedies prescribed. A review and revision of these factors appear indicated to refute previously held concepts and bring some order to this ubiquitous condition; hence, this presentation that clears the air.

Low back disorder is considered a more appropriate term even though the symptom of "pain" may be the factor that brings the patient to the physician; it is functional disorder that merits attention and its remedy.

Disorder is defined as a "Pathological condition of the mind and body" (1) . . . "A disturbance of the normal state of the body" (2). Disorder of the functional anatomical aspect of the low back is important, but it is only one aspect of the disorder that now must be considered and addressed.

The clinical biomechanics of the spine have been well documented and problems of management have also been well discussed, but it is difficult for the average physician to remain current with what is significantly pertinent or effective. The manner in which impaired biomechanics cause the symptoms of impairment also needs clarification.

Recent literature has uncovered many factors that include "stability" of the spine, and current literature has now made understanding this condition attainable (3).

The numerous articles regarding "pain" also pose problems of applicability as to which tissue changes are responsible. A recent concept based on the original works of Cannon and Rosenblueth's Law of Denervation (4) has promoted early recognition of low back disorders and may even clarify the physiologic basis for chiropractic manipulation, acupuncture, and other physical modalities. It presents a basis for use of various medications as well as modalities.

Because pain does remain a significant factor as causation of impairment, it receives review of all recent investigations and application of medications in the literature.

With low back disorders being so prevalent and costly to society, a review of these current findings justifies this update. The increasing incidence of chronicity developing from inappropriately addressed management of the acute impairment merits discussion, which is a failure in more recent publications regarding the low back.

Low Back Disorders addresses the recent studies and applications of these factors with the hope that future impaired patients may benefit.

Rene Cailliet, M.D.

REFERENCES

1. Thomas CL. *Taber's Cyclopedic Medical Dictionary,* 16th Edition. Philadelphia: F. A. Davis, 1989.
2. Brown L, ed. *The New Shorter Oxford English Dictionary.* Oxford: Clarendon Press, 1993.
3. Richardson C, Jull G, Hodges P, Hides J. *Therapeutic Exercise For Spinal Segmental Stabilization in Low Back Pain.* Edinburgh: Churchill Livingstone, 1999.
4. Gunn CC. *The Gunn Approach to the Treatment of Chronic Pain.* New York: Churchill Livingstone, 1989.

1. THE CURRENT CONCERN WITH THE LOW BACK

Prevalence is a useful measure of the extent of a problem. Prevalence measures how many persons have the problem at any given time. As compared with cancer, AIDS, and cardiovascular malfunction, the low back has gained major interest because of its prevalence as measured by the cost to society, cost to industry, and effect on the quality of life (1,2).

DIAGNOSIS

Despite all the research and clinical experience in the diagnosis and treatment of low back disorders (LBDs), there has been little significant progress in understanding the mechanisms of the low back and its management (3,4). This has inevitably led to considering LBDs as psychosocial rather than as mechanical in their causation and has therefore affected understanding them.

A meaningful pathoanatomic diagnosis is rare and at best strictly subjective. This must be kept in mind before undertaking expensive, prolonged treatment (5).

A history as elicited by the examiner is the patient's narrative of the event and the problem. The history is guided by questions from the examiner to clarify the precise symptoms, their site, severity, and reason for occurrence. ("In the mind of the patient what was the reason for the cause of the problem and its subsequent disability." [5])

The patient must furnish all these pertinent factors just as he or she furnishes the examiner with his or her mechanical, psychologic, and socioeconomic concerns. The examiner must determine what these complaints mean to the person as to the effect on his or her life-style, economic future, and expectations from any proposed treatments.

The patient expresses the incurred disability in the history. The impairment must be ascertained from the physical examination to determine the "diagnosis" of the impairment. *Diagnosis* has been defined as, "The process of determining the nature of a disease . . . from the patient's symptoms . . . a conclusion that ascertains the cause of mechanical" (6). This definition assumes that low back complaints are a "disease," which is defined literally as "the lack of ease: a pathologic condition of the body that presents a group of clinical signs and symptoms, and laboratory findings, peculiar to it and that sets the condition apart as an abnormal entity differing from other normal or pathologic body states" (6).

The concept of disease may include the condition of illness or suffering not necessarily arising from pathologic changes in the body. There is a major distinction between disease and illness in that the former is usually tangible and may even be measured, whereas illness is highly individual and personal, as with pain, suffering, and distress. "A person may be extremely ill, as with hysteria or mental illness, but have no evidence of disease as measured by pathologic changes in the body" (7).

A precise diagnosis of a low back impairment is handicapped by lack of reliable objective findings (8), presenting the "enigma" of the title of this text.

Impairment has been defined by the World Health Organization, American Medical Association, and Social Security guidelines (9–11) as "any loss or abnormality of psychologic, physiologic or anatomic structure or 'function' . . . leading to loss of normal bodily function." Social Security guidelines (12) define *impairment* as "being demonstrable by medically acceptable clinical and laboratory diagnostic techniques." Simplistically, *impairment* is "observable and determinable loss of function from structural bodily elements" and *disability* is "subjective inability to function in activities of daily living." What the patient cannot do because of pain is the subjective evaluation of disability.

A meaningful history must reveal what movements, positions, and activities cause or aggravate the subjective complaints, as this is very important in informing the examiner of the tissue site of the impairment and also informs the examiner about the mechanical basis of the functional impairment and what the patient considers as pertinent and causative (13,14).

The possibility of recurrence or aggravation by an activity has become a significant concern of the patient, which is why the patient must understand the activity that may have caused the impairment and avoid or modify it in the future. The examiner must also ascertain the specific activity.

Fear–avoidance is a major factor in the development and maintenance of chronic musculoskeletal pain, impairment, and disability (15). In the acute phase, where pain is aggravated by certain movement and activities, these are understandably avoided, but when avoidance of all activity is prolonged, it may lead to muscle weakness and fear.

What these activities are, in the mind of the patient, is important to ascertain, as they will be important in treatment and prognosis.

SYMPTOMS RELATED TO THE LOW BACK

Pain is usually the major reason for the patient seeking relief and reassurance, so this symptom must be addressed even though the precise cause is unknown initially. Impairment and disability ultimately become the major concern while the precise tissue causing pain is ascertained.

Patients perceive pain differently. The International Association for the Study of Pain has wisely defined *pain* as "an unpleasant sensory and 'emotional' experience associated with actual or perceived tissue damage" (16). Pain is always a personal experience; no one can really feel another's pain. There are no objective measurements of pain, so the patient, and ultimately the examiner, must ascertain the basis, significance, and consequence of this symptom.

How and why the symptom of pain affects function must also be elicited in the history, as the functional loss claimed by the patient and subjectively elicited by the examiner from the history attempts to determine the "disability." The objective of the subsequent examination therefore becomes the finding of the specific tissue in the low back. It is hoped that the tissue site of the symptoms is determined by the specific movement or activity that initiates the specific symptom.

How the pain impairs function is the most significant aspect of the examination. This is often very difficult for the patient to express, as the focus is on the subjective basis of the symptoms and not necessarily on the structural basis of the injured tissue and its implication.

As the interpretation of low back impairment has been considered to be mechanical (14), specific tissues within the low back have been identified and have become the concentration of the examiner and ultimately the concern of the patient. These tissues are, in the concept of the author, the "end organs" of the neurologic sequence (Fig. 1.0) and must be addressed in the examination.

The phrase "I was hurt" is rarely accurate. Usually what has occurred is "I hurt myself by doing. . . ." This statement is probably more accurate. The neuromuscular phase of the neurologic sequence described (Fig. 1.1) does not refute that a specific tissue has been traumatized by inappropriate movement. It means that a specific tissue in the low back has been traumatized. The how becomes more important in understanding how misuse of the normal function has caused the impairment and thus the symptoms.

The tissue sites within the functional unit that may be sites of nociception have been well established. They are:

1. External fibers of the intervertebral disc
2. Posterior longitudinal ligament
3. Nerve root dural sheath
4. Synovial capsule of the facets
5. Ligaments: interspinous or supraspinous
6. Erector spinae muscles
7. Fascia of the muscles

The basis of a meaningful examination is to determine which of these tissue sites are the sites of the patient's symptoms and the basis of impairment and subsequent disability. The history has been elicited to establish the basis, determining how that injury occurred so that it does not happen again.

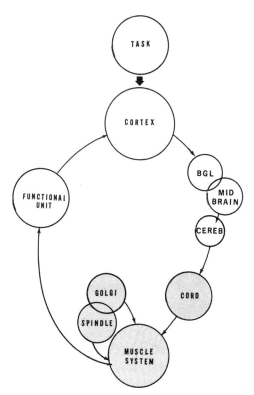

FIG. 1.0. The task intended initiates "patterns" of neuromuscular activities that end in its completion by the "end organs": the discs, facets, ligaments, and muscles. The "patterns" are ingrained in the cortex and are modified with practice and repetition. The "patterns" are coordinated within the mid-brain, basal ganglia (BGL) and the cerebellum (CEREB) and are transmitted through the spinal cord to the muscular system. The muscular system is coordinated by its intrinsic system of Golgi apparatus and spindle cells to activate the functional unit.

It can be summarized in the evolution of LBDs that faulty biomechanical function has caused damage to a tissue of the low back that is known to be a site of nociception: the intervertebral disc, the facets, the muscles, and/or the ligaments of the low back.

The low back must have stability, yet that term is not well defined. *Instability* has been defined by White and Panjabi (15) as "the loss of the ability of the spine under physiologic loads to maintain its pattern of displacement so there are no initial or additional neurologic deficits, no major deformity and no incapacitating pain." How this definition is used clinically remains unclear (16). The hypothesis is that the spine as a structure has lost some of its mechanical integrity through some form of soft-tissue compromise. Diagnostic and assessment techniques are not currently well developed.

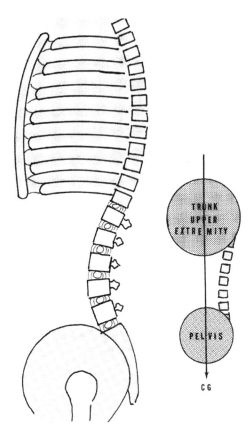

FIG. 1.1. The ligamentous spine. The lumbosacral spine basically supports two inflexible systems: the thoracic spine, made inflexible by the attachments of the ribs, and the pelvis, which articulates between two femoral heads. The figure to the right shows the stability of the two segments balanced by the flexible rod: the lumbosacral spine. CG, center of gravity.

The lumbosacral spine, the low back, (Fig. 1.1) typically contains five lumbar "functional units" that contain two vertebra, the intervertebral disc, long ligaments, posterior facets (zygapophyseal joints), and the back muscles. The ligamentous spine, which excludes the back muscles, is considered unstable in that it cannot support half of the total body weight.

In the upright posture the lumbar spine structurally supports the axial compressive forces from the loads of the thorax, head, and cervical spine; the upper extremities; and any load the extremities may hold, and do so at a distance from the center of gravity.

It is apparent that the muscular system is mandatory to afford stability of the ligamentous low back. This will be discussed in detail in subsequent chapters. All the tissues contained within the functional unit contribute to the stability and when impaired by faulty function therefore also contribute to impairment and disability.

SPECIFIC TISSUE OF THE LOW BACK: SITES OF NOCICEPTION
As the purpose of the examination is to determine the tissue site as well as the mechanism by which injury has occurred, each tissue within the low back must be considered.

The Intervertebral Disc
The intervertebral discs by their hydrodynamic structure function to maintain specific distance of the two adjacent vertebra and permit motion known as rotation (10 degrees) and translation (4 mm) (Fig. 1.2).

The collagen fibers of the normal disc (Fig. 1.3) allow normal physiologic elongation and recovery but excessive and unphysiologic motion of the functional unit, especially rotation damage the annular fibers. Disruption of the annular container allows the nucleus centrally located to herniate outward through the disrupted annular fibers. This "herniation" is the outward bulging of the nucleus, which then may encroach on the sensitive posterior longitudinal ligament and the dorsal root ganglion and its dural sheath within the foramen. Tearing of the annular fibers liberates nociceptive chemicals of the matrix, which become inflammatory (Fig. 1.4).

It has been postulated that pain "in" the low back and radicular pain "from" the back occurs as a chemical as well as a mechanical compression of herniated disc material to the nerve root components, including the dural sheath. The pathomechanics remain unclear.

Among the chemicals released from the herniated disc are biologically active proteoglycans released from the nucleus pulposus that may irritate the nerve roots and the posterior longitudinal ligament. Phospholipid A2 has been postulated as playing a major role in pain from herniated lumbar disc material.

Examination of disc material removed surgically has revealed that after disc injury an infiltration of inflammatory cells occurs,

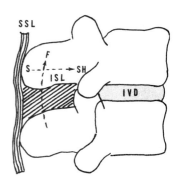

FIG. 1.2. Rotation and translation of a functional unit. A functional unit is shown where rotation (F flexion) is possible to 10 degrees and translation (S-SH) is physiologically possible to 10 mm. ISL, interspinous ligament; IVD, intervertebral disc; SSL, supraspinatus ligament.

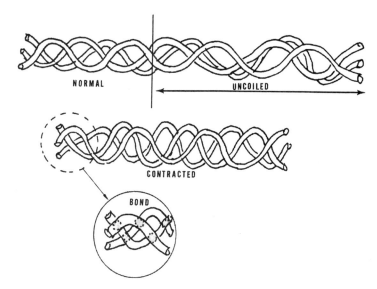

FIG. 1.3. A collagen fiber. A collagen fiber is a trihelix of amino acids in chains that intertwine. Each fibril has a physiologic curvature that elongates by uncurling and recurling when the elongating force is removed. The chains are bonded at each intersection.

such as macrophages, lymphocytes, and fibroblasts, as well as production of prostaglandin E2, thromboxane B2, leukotriene B4, and nitric oxide.

Recently, it has been proposed that cytokines and chemokines also play a role in chemical pathomechanism of radicular pain (17). In herniated disc tissue increased levels of tumor necrosis factor

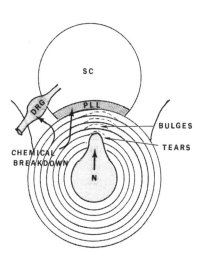

FIG. 1.4. Internal herniation of the nucleus. Tears in the outer annulus permit the nucleus (N) to herniate outward (*arrow*) toward the posterior longitudinal ligament (PLL) or the dorsal root ganglion (DRG); both are sensitive. The chemical breakdown of the matrix is an inflammatory substance. SC, spinal canal.

(TNF)-alpha, interleukin (IL)-1,1 IL-6, and granulocyte-macrophage colony stimulating factor (GM-CSF), all inflammatory cytokines, have been found.

Inflammatory cytokines are primarily related to defense against tissue inflammation (18). Chemokines help control the influx of inflammatory cells such as neutrophils, macrophages, and lymphocytes into the tissue sites and are critical in producing chronic inflammation. Their role in inflammation from herniated discs remains unclear, but IL-8 appears to be involved in producing radicular pain.

The presence in recent discoveries of cytokines and chemokines in low back and radicular disorders provides a target for therapeutic intervention (17).

FACTORS OF EXAMINATION TO DETERMINE THE PATHOANATOMIC BASIS OF SYMPTOMS

The pathoanatomic factors of a LBD demand performing a meaningful examination. This begins by observing the demeanor of the patient and the expression of pain by facial expression and the choice of words that indicate the severity and its relationship to disability (19).

The movements of the patient—including gait, seating posture, and manner of response to the requested activities must be observed—as they depict which movements are causative and therefore avoided by the patient.

Evaluating the way the patient walks is important, but gait is complex and may be influenced by the guarded motions imposed by the patient's reaction to the painful low back (20). Abnormal gait may be a sequela of impairment from neurologic loss resulting from low back impairment and nerve root entrapment.

When sitting presents a problem, the sitting posture must be evaluated. Sitting normally causes the spine to assume a flexed (kyphotic posture) with an erect centralized position. These positions place mechanical stress on the intervertebral discs, facets, ligaments, and low back extensor muscles, so that all these tissues must be evaluated in subsequent portions of the examination.

The history must have revealed which movements the patient considered to have initiated the onset of low back pain and which movements, activities, and positions currently initiate or aggravate the pain. A very important part of the subsequent physical examination is to reproduce the alleged pain by actively and passively placing the patient through various positions, activities, and movements and reproducing the pain. By reproducing the pain claimed by the patient, not only the tissue involved but also the mechanism of the impairment can be deduced. Its explanation to the patient, in understandable terms and illustrations, becomes not only the basis but the crucial element to meaningful therapeutic intervention and patient cooperation.

TISSUE SITES OF PAIN AND IMPAIRMENT

Returning to the concept of the end organ in the neurologic sequence being the pathoanatomic tissue sites that causes the subjective symptoms, we must now establish how this tissue causes the impairment. These end organs, which are vital for normal function, are also innervated by nociceptive nerve fibers and thus can be the sites of pain production.

The following end-organ tissues ascertained as being sites of nociception are the intervertebral disc, the facets, the facet capsules, the erector spinae muscles, and the nerve root dural sleeves. Each will be discussed with regard to their normal function, their impairment, and their role in producing nociception.

THE INTERVERTEBRAL DISC

The intervertebral disc has become the *bête noire* of low back pain since the classic work of Mixter and Barr in the 1930s (21). This hydrodynamic avascular soft tissue that separates the vertebrae and affords support yet permits motion between the vertebra has been extensively studied in terms of not only structure and function but also pathology.

Gravity affects the disc, as does muscular contraction. In an average day approximately 3% to 10% of the disc fluid is normally lost. It requires 10 hours for total loss of fluid and 2 hours for recovery (22). As the tissue is avascular, recovery and nutrition have been determined to be via imbibition from the surrounding blood vessels that are present in the subchondral tissues of the vertebrae. To ensure more vascular supply of nutrition to the disc, cyclic loading and unloading must occur, the latter for sufficiently long periods and the former for brief periods.

Review of the voluminous medical literature implies that the forces needed to damage the disc annular fibers must be excessive torque and shear combined with excessive compression. This not only damages the annular fibers but also disrupts the integrity of the matrix, a mucopolysaccharide with negative polarity, causing it to lose its ability to imbibe water and maintain its hydrodynamic force.

To incriminate the disc as the site of impairment, and of pain, the history must indicate the precise mechanism that may have caused damage to the disc structure; thus a torque force, probably with compression, must be surmised. In taking a meaningful history, the examiner must recall the specific movement that the patient probably made at the time of the injury and what activity was intended.

The specific movement inquiry must ascertain whether the person was bending, twisting, or lifting, and the distance of the object to one side. All this information will ensure the determination of the precise mechanism that may have damaged the disc.

The examiner must inquire as to the patient's state of mind at the time of injury: whether there was impatience, fatigue, anger, or boredom. These will help determine the speed and accuracy of action, as distraction impairs proper neuromusculoskeletal function.

The annular fibers of the disc are composed of collagen that have limited elongation before disruption. Disruption occurs when the fibers are stretched beyond their physiologic limits. Disruption may also occur when the forces cause the annular fibers to be torn from their site of attachment to the vertebral plate. With either mechanism the specific significant force must be deduced from the history.

Low back pain, without radicular symptoms, must be assumed to be attributable to disc pathology that has encroached on the posterior longitudinal ligament. The resultant symptoms from compression on the sensitive posterior longitudinal ligament are exclusively related to the low back and not to the lower extremities. Pain from a central disc herniation is usually noted in the midline of the low back. It may be noted without movement but is particularly elicited from lumbar flexion, as trunk flexion allegedly protrudes the disc nucleus posteriorly and thus against the posterior longitudinal ligament.

Symptoms and impairment are considered to be caused by discogenic pathology from the history and findings of pain located in the middle low back, a limited range of motion due to muscle contraction termed *spasm,* and low back muscle tenderness. None of these findings specifically indicate the disc as the source of pain and impairment but are merely suggestive (23,24) (Fig. 1.5).

Other tests and clinical signs are needed to confirm that the intervertebral disc is the cause of the symptoms and findings; as of today they are often inconclusive.

SPINAL INSTABILITY
When spinal instability is considered a pertinent factor in low back pain, accurate clinical testing is difficult without radiologic confirmation.

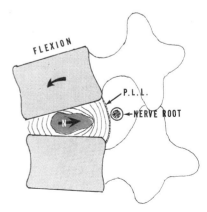

FIG. 1.5. Disc protrusion from lumbar flexion. As there is flexion in a functional unit, the nucleus (N) presses the posterior annular fibers and encroach on the posterior longitudinal ligament (PLL). The nerve roots are located laterally and may not be encroached on.

An "instability test" has been postulated in which the patient is placed in the prone position and the examiner's thumb finds the interspinous space and exerts downward pressure, seeking a reproduction of pain by mechanically moving the vertebra on its adjacent vertebra.

Several spaces are identified and tested. If none are found to be sensitive, the remainder of the test cannot be performed. If a segment is found to be sensitive the patient is asked to elevate the head and shoulders, creating active spinal muscular contraction, and the test is performed again. The test is only "positive" if pain also occurs in the relaxed prone position; muscular contraction suggests paravertebral muscle involvement (Fig. 1.6).

A "weight relief test" also implies discogenic causation when the supine patient with hips and knees flexed has the legs elevated. This flexes the low back passively and is considered "positive" if pain is diminished.

RADICULAR SYMPTOMS AND FINDINGS

The presence of leg pain as well as low back pain enhances a more specific diagnosis of discogenic pain, indicating increased discogenic pressure and chemical irritation of the nerve root in the foramen or spinal canal. Any action that increases intradiscal pressure is suggestive of discogenic etiology of low back disorder. Intradiscal pressure is higher when sitting than when standing and is elevated when bending forward, bending to the side, lifting, straining, coughing, or

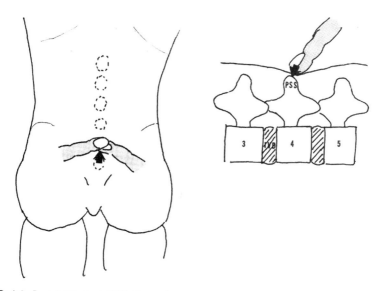

FIG. 1.6. Instability test. With the patient prone the examiner manually identifies the sensitive disc space then transmits a direct force. Eliciting pain is a "positive" test.

sneezing (25,26). Any or all of these may be elicited in the patient's history (25,26).

Leg pain, with or without low back pain, but usually with the former, is considered discogenic "straight-leg raising" (also termed Laseque's test or sciatic stretch test) is positive. It must be performed accurately and must be consistently positive if it is to provide reliable evaluative results (27–29).

The straight-leg-raising (SLR) test involves reproducing the pain by gradually elevating the straight leg (extended knee), then lowering it a few degrees to diminish the pain, which then must be aggravated by dorsiflexing the foot–ankle or flexing the head–neck (Fig. 1.7).

In doing the SLR test it must be determined whether the elicited pain is muscular or neurologic, as both will elicit similar pain from the procedure. The confusion in terminology was highlighted by Akkerveeken (30,31), who attempted to differentiate *radicular pain* from *sciatica*. The former should be used for patients suffering from pain resulting from pathology of the spinal nerve root, whereas the latter is a neuralgia of the sciatic nerve trunk.

The term *sciatica* was derived from the Latin *ischialgia*, meaning "pain [*algia*] in the lower buttocks region [*ischia*]." Hippocrates (32) called this type of pain "hip pain," but in 1770 Cotugno (33) differentiated hip pain from pain noted in the hip region from sciatic nerve involvement. Differentiation of sciatica as a neuritis from neuralgia resulting from nerve root irritation was postulated by Wertheim-Salomonson (34). Verbiest (35) postulated that pain resulted from compression of a nerve root because of irritation of the nervi nervosum of the root sheath when the pain was eliminated by placing a drop of cocaine on the sheath.

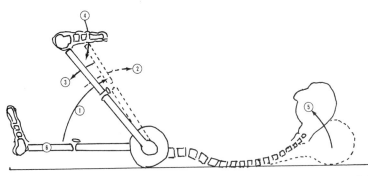

FIG. 1.7. Straight-leg-raising test. With the patient supine the leg is raised with knee extended (1) until pain is experienced (2); then the leg is descended (3) and the foot-ankle is dorsiflexed (4). As confirmation, the head and neck are flexed (5). Pain from (4,5) confirms a "positive straight leg test"; (6) is the dependent other leg that stabilizes the pelvis.

The concept of pain as due to the nerve root and/or dural compression is now challenged, as acute compression of a nerve is usually painless, whereas compression of an "inflamed" dorsal root ganglion causes ectopic nerve root firing (36,37). Vibration has also been considered as a cause of ectopic firing.

Recent research has implicated the dorsal root ganglion as a modulator of low back pain (37), but compression has been questioned. A further enigma has recently arisen when it was found that application of autologous nucleus pulposus (herniated material from the same source) to the nerve root reduces the blood flow in the dorsal root ganglion from intraneural edema but does not "clarify which of these changes caused symptoms of the lower extremity" (38).

This decreased blood flow and intraneural edema of the nerve root and DRG (dorsal root ganglion) also caused a thermal deficit of the lower extremity, implicating an involvement of the sympathetic nervous system and not merely a chemical involvement of the somatic nervous system. The dermatomal areas reveal a decrease in local temperature. Ectopic firing in the dorsal root ganglion and increased sympathetic activity causing vasoconstriction through a somatosympathetic reflex present another enigma in understanding radicular pain.

The dorsal root has been implicated as a modulator of low back pain (37). The dorsal root is considered a vital link between the internal and external environment and the spinal cord. The primary sensory role of the cord is to receive afferent stimuli in the form of action potentials and relay these impulses to the brain.

In discogenic pathology, with no leg pains or lower-extremity findings, the SLR test, causing more low back pain than leg pain, is considered to be due to increased intradiscal pressure against the posterior longitudinal ligament. A "flip" test then may be diagnostic of discogenic etiology. In performing this test the patient is seated with the calves against the edge of the table and the hands on the edge of the table; then the flexed knee is straightened to full extension. When this maneuver causes more low back pain than leg pain, the test is considered positive (Fig. 1.8).

CONFIRMATORY TESTS

Myelography, CT discography, or MRI studies may confirm the presence of disc herniation and protrusion into the spinal canal with pressure on the posterior longitudinal ligament or of encroachment on the nerve root at the specific level and side elicited by the examination.

MYOGENIC LOW BACK PAIN

The history of a patient with low back pain that suggests a myogenic basis indicates that the erector spinae muscles have been misused or overused. It must be remembered that discogenic low back pain is

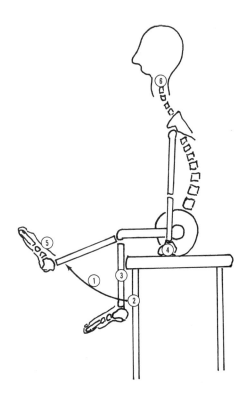

FIG. 1.8. "Flip test." With the patient seated on a table and legs against that table (2) the leg is elevated until pain is elicited. The other leg is dependent (3) and the patient supporting his body with his hands against the table (4). The ankle (5) may be dorsiflexed to accentuate the test, and nuchal flexion can be used (6).

complicated by simultaneous muscle reaction and pain and that muscular contraction also increases discogenic pressure.

Several diagnostic factors implicate low back pain as being myogenic:

1. There is local tenderness.
2. Pain is reproduced by passive stretching.
3. Pain is aggravated by isolated muscle contraction against resistance.
4. Tenderness is predominantly in the paravertebral muscles just lateral to the midline.

There is also frequently tenderness of the gluteus maximus. There are currently no diagnostic tests that confirm myogenic pain. The diagnosis is exclusively clinical.

TENSION MYOSITIS SYNDROME

In his classic text Sarno (39) postulates that most, if not all, low back pain is caused by tension myositis syndrome (TMS), with the tension in the muscles being related to deep-seated emotional tension with the muscles (back muscles in this case) being the external manifestation of deep-seated and repressed emotional problems.

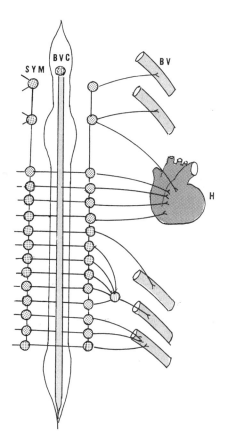

FIG. 1.9. Sympathetic nervous system control of the circulation. The autonomic nervous system (SYM) controls the vasomotor system: the blood vessels (BV) and the heart (H). At the upper aspect of the cord resides the vasomotor center (BVC).

This is a provocative concept with significant neurophysiologic confirmation (40). In this concept, localized ischemia of the muscles from vasomotor contraction resulting from deep-seated emotional stresses causes pain and limited motion (Figs. 1.9–1.12).

This concept has received wide acceptance and brought apparent benefit to patients who accept it and undergo appropriate treatment. Such a concept can be accepted, but Sarno goes further and states that there is no mechanical basis for low back pain, which is contrary to current literature.

The concept of TMS is acceptable if this tension is implied as adversely affecting normal mechanical factors of back function leading to pain and impairment. Further discussion will ensue in the section on treatment.

Examination for TMS reveals localized tenderness over the affected muscle from digital pressure. In the presence of TMS, tenderness also occurs over other muscles than those of the low back. Table 1.1 lists these sites (41).

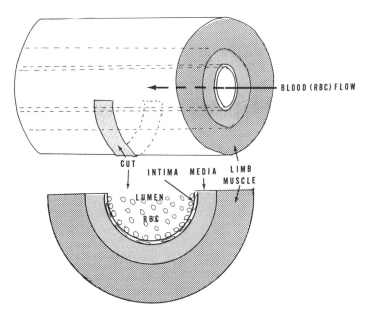

FIG. 1.10. Control of arterial lumen. A lateral view of an artery with its lumen, surrounded by the intima, then the media, and ultimately the adventitia and surrounding muscles. As muscles contract they constrict the lumen and decrease blood flow.

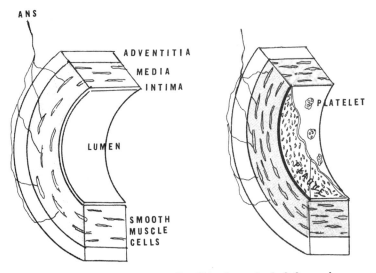

FIG. 1.11. Control of the muscular media of blood vessels. Left figure shows normal control of the three layers of blood vessels. Excessive prolonged autonomic impulses cause constriction of the media with ultimate thickening and narrowing of the lumen. Prolonged constriction of blood flow can cause platelets to form plaques within the lumen.

GOOD   BAD

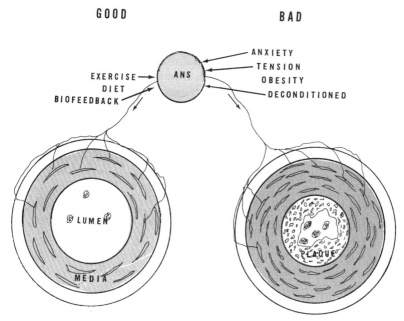

FIG. 1.12. Good and bad effect of autonomic control of blood vessels. The autonomic nervous system (ANS) favorably dilates blood vessels from exercise and appropriate diet. Anxiety, tension, obesity, and deconditioning unfavorably affect blood vessels, with ultimate atherosclerosis and plaque formation.

Numerous areas of muscle tenderness other than the low back imply the presence of generalized TMS as the basis for the localized tenderness. Many patients report having pain for the first few hours of the day, then relief from activity. Others do the opposite: no pain early in the day but increased as the day progresses. Pain is often chronic and usually there is no relief from many of the accepted procedures and modalities other than the application of heat.

Examination requires deep digital pressure over the areas identified by the patient and reproducing the specific pain or at least tenderness over the site of the pain. What makes TMS probable as a system

TABLE 1.1. TENDERNESS ON PALPATION IN TMS PATIENTS

Buttock, 60%
Shoulder, 12%
Neck, 9%
Lumbar, 8%
Thoracic, 7%
Other, 4%

Reproduced from Sarno J. *Mind over back pain.* New York: William Morrow, 1984:74.

status is that areas other than those producing low back pain are also palpably tender.

Muscular pain, besides being considered as the result of ischemia, may have a direct route and be mediated via the ventral (motor) nerve. Nerve roots that are allegedly primarily if not exclusively considered motor were suggested to be sensory by Frykholm (40) when he caused pain by electrically stimulating ventral nerve roots, then relieving the pain by blocking these nerves with cocaine. This finding implicates muscles as a potential site of nociception.

FACET ETIOLOGY OF LOW BACK PAIN

Low back pain occurring from facet pathology is suspected when local low back pain occurs from active and passive extension of the low back and is aggravated by simultaneous ipsilateral side bending. There is local tenderness over the facet (42). Chapter 4 gives a full discussion of facet pathology.

SPINAL STENOSIS

Spinal stenosis is suspected when there is a history of pseudoclaudication. Because pseudoclaudication accompanies facet arthrosis and discogenic disease, both of these are revealed in the history and physical findings. The history and confirmation by radiologic studies generally make the diagnosis of spinal stenosis.

The pseudoclaudication history is one of low back and leg pain that comes on after a period of walking and that is relieved by ceasing walking and assuming a trunk-flexed posture such as bending forward or sitting. Pain noted in the leg is usually unilateral and is accompanied by the sensation of numbness and weakness in dermatomal and myotomal areas of the leg. Relief of pain also occurs from the patient sitting, leaning forward, or lying down. Symptoms that change when there is a change in posture, extension to flexion, are diagnostic.

A Phalen-like test for spinal stenosis is to reproduce symptoms (leg pain, weakness, and/or numbness) by having the patient stand upright and then bend backward and sustain that posture for a full minute or longer. This position increases the stenosis. Relief is initiated by having the patient assume a forward flexed posture for several minutes. The final diagnosis is from imaging confirmation tests.

NEUROLOGIC DETERMINATION OF NERVE ROOT INVOLVEMENT

In determining which nerve root is involved and responsible for the radiating pain from the lumbosacral plexus, a careful neurologic examination is diagnostic. Sensory testing by touch, pin scratch, cotton wisps, or tuning fork will determine the root level (Fig. 1.13). Motor testing of a specific muscle to determine its myotome root level is done by manually resisting and measuring the strength and endurance by repetitive contraction of that muscle. As the nerves of the lumbosacral plexus include all the nerve roots from L1 to S1, each muscle of the

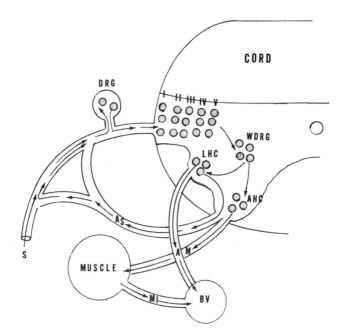

FIG. 1.13. Composition of a nerve root. A typical nerve root contains the following: Sensory fiber (S) enters the dorsal root ganglion (DRG), then the gray matter of the cord, into Rexed layers I, II, III, IV, and V. There is a connection with the wide dynamic range ganglia (WDRG) with internuncial connections to the lateral horn cells (LHC) and the anterior horn cells (AHC). The AHC (motor M) fibers go to specific muscles. The sympathetic fibers (A) emanating from the LHC go to blood vessels (BV) and are sensory (AS).

lower extremity must be tested and the opposite (contralateral) muscle tested for comparison.

The S1 root supplies the gastrocnemius soleus muscle and hence can be tested by having the patient stand on one leg and arise repeatedly for several elevations to determine strength and endurance. A mildly involved nerve root lesion may permit a few contractions but fail to allow repeated elevations. The other leg is so tested for comparison. The S1 myotome can also be evaluated by testing the strength of the gluteus maximus. This is done by having the patient assume the supine position on an examining table, flexing the leg to 90 degrees, and with that foot on the table elevating the pelvis repeatedly. The other leg is similarly tested (Fig. 1.14).

The S1 myotome can also be evaluated by testing the hamstring muscle. With the patient seated. The L4 dermatome is the area of the inner aspect of the lower leg. With S1, L5, and L4 nerve root involvement the Laseque SLR test is positive, but it is not positive in higher nerve root entrapments. The L3 myotome is to the quadriceps muscles

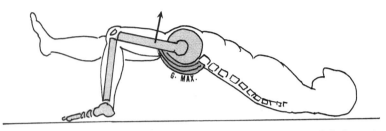

FIG. 1.14. Testing the S1 myotome by testing the gluteus maximus. With the patient in the supine position and the knee flexed to a right angle, the pelvis is elevated repeatedly to test strength and endurance. The other leg is similarly tested.

and the dermatomal area is to the posterior thigh and anterior knee regions. The knee jerk reflex designates the L3–L4 nerve roots. The SLR is not positive but the stretch test of the femoral nerve is. The femoral nerve stretch test is performed with the patient prone and the leg flexed. As the foot approaches the buttocks there is pain in the anterior thigh area that is not experienced in the other leg (Fig. 1.15).

CLINICAL MEASUREMENT OF MUSCLE FUNCTION

As the control of the vertebral function is totally dependent on appropriate muscle function, this motor function should be evaluated for both stabilization and kinetic action. Unfortunately, this measurement testing remains ineffective. There is a lack of physical outcome parameters that are valid, precise, sensitive, and clinically relevant (43).

The muscles that are deficient in motor function are deep in the trunk, close to the vertebrae, and not readily visible or accessible to examination. Traditional muscle testing of more peripheral muscles involved in trunk function are not the muscles that lend stability to the vertebral column. These muscles, the transversus abdominis and multifidus, usually contract in isometric low-level contraction independently of the global muscles that activate the spine.

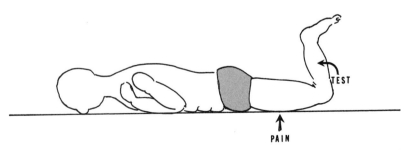

FIG. 1.15. Femoral stretch test. With the patient in the prone position the knee is flexed, and as the foot approaches the buttocks, pain occurs in the anterior thigh area.

To test these stabilizing muscles, have the patient draw in the abdominal wall and hold this position for 10 or more seconds. These muscles must be activated without contraction of the global muscles (Fig. 1.16).

Testing the segmental multifidus muscles is also necessary, albeit difficult. In the prone position the examiner deeply palpates the muscles on the paravertebral lumbar spine adjacent to the vertebrae. In this prone position the patient is asked to "swell the muscle under the superficial abdominal muscles." This may require some training of the patient. Proper pelvic tilting is also a test for the deep stabilizing muscles.

TEST OF AN INCREASE IN INTRATHECAL PRESSURE

An increase in intrathecal pressure (revealed by the history) that accentuates the radicular pain can be tested by methods that increase intrathecal pressure. Several tests can be used.

The Milgram Test

With the patient lying supine on the examining table both legs are slightly elevated by the patient and held there for 30 seconds. If radicular pain occurs the test is considered positive. In the presence of weak abdominal muscles this maneuver may cause hyperextension of the lumbar lordosis that causes low back pain. This differentiation must be clinically defined (Fig. 1.17).

The Naffziger Test

Increase in intrathecal pressure can be caused by compressing the jugular veins in the neck for approximately 10 seconds until the patient's face becomes flush. During the jugular compression the patient is asked to cough. A positive test is not specifically diagnostic of a herniated disc, as it is also present in other cord compression syndromes. It is not considered a routine test for lumbar disc herniation but, at best, is confirmation of nerve root compression.

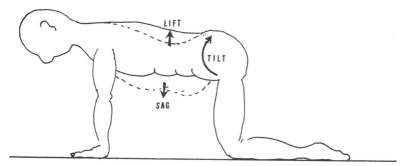

FIG. 1.16. "Drawing in" deep muscle testing. In a four-point kneeling position the patient elevates the lower back and holds it there for more than 10 seconds.

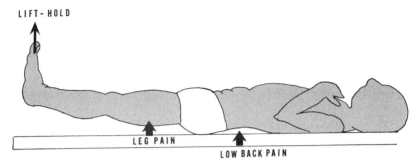

FIG. 1.17. Milgram test. The patient actively raises both legs approximately 3 inches from the table and holds them there for approximately 30 seconds. If pain radiates down the leg, the test is considered positive.

The Valsalva Maneuver

Leg radiating pain caused or aggravated by bearing down as in straining for bowel or bladder evacuation or during cough or sneeze suggests dural nerve compression. This test is essentially performed by taking a careful history and specifically asking the patient to bear down while holding the breath. The test is not specific for discogenic disease but is merely a test of increased intrathecal pressure.

The Kernig Test

Forcefully flexing the head and neck causes a stretching of the dural sheath and is similar to the SLR test with simultaneous ankle dorsiflexion. Radicular pain from this maneuver is considered positive.

ELECTROMYOGRAPHY

When there is subjective and objective evidence of nerve root entrapment an electromyographic test can confirm objective evidence of this neuropathy and accurately designate the precise disc level.

DISCOGRAPHY

Injection of a radiopaque material into the nucleus of the disc has been advocated as designating the presence of disc herniation and specifying the precise identification of which disc is involved (44). Reproduction of the pain also is considered to confirm that a herniated disc is responsible for the patient's pain.

An appropriate examination, a careful meaningful history, and confirmation by diagnostic radiologic studies should determine the presence and cause of the patient's symptoms and findings.

SUMMARY

A meaningful examination to determine objective findings that confirm what has been stated in the history demands full knowledge of functional anatomy and a recognition of the deviations that were elicited from the examination. The tendency to attribute all symptoms and their pathoanatomy to confirmatory tests is to be discouraged. These tests merely clarify the results of the clinical tests performed by the examiner. Giving these tests a label is only accepted if the true meaning of that label is understood and given to the patient.

REFERENCES

1. Walker BF. The prevalence of low back pain: a systematic review of the literature from 1966 to 1998. *J Spinal Disorders* 2000;13:205–217.
2. Bombardier C, Baldwin J-A, Crull L. The epidemiology of regional musculo-skeletal disorders: Canada. In: Hadler NM, ed. *Arthritis and society.* London: Butterworths, 1985:104–118.
3. Bigos S, Barrice M. The impact of spinal disorders in industry. In: Frymoyer JW, ed. *The adult spine: principles and practice,* 2nd ed. Philadelphia: Lippincott-Raven, 1997:151–1161
4. Teasell R, Harth M. Functional restoration. Returning patients with chronic low back pain to work: revolution or fad? *Spine* 996:21:844–847.
5. Dillane J, Fry J, Kalton G. Acute back syndrome: a study from general practice. *BMJ* 1996:2:82–84
6. Brown L, ed. *The new shorter Oxford English dictionary.* Oxford: Clarendon Press, 1993.
7. Thomas CL, ed. *Taber's cyclopedic medical dictionary,* 16th ed. Philadelphia: FA Davis, 1989.
8. Laros GS. Differential diagnosis of low back pain. In: Mayer TG, Mooney V, Gatchel RJ, eds. *Contemporary conservative care for painful spinal disorders,* Philadelphia: Lea & Febiger, 1991.
9. World Health Organization. *International classification of impairments, disabilities and handicaps.* Geneva: World Health Organization, 1980.
10. American Medical Association. Guides to the evaluation of permanent impairments of the extremities and back. *JAMA* 1958;66(Suppl):1.
11. U.S. Bureau of Disability Insurance. *Disability evaluation under Social Security: a handbook for physicians.* Washington, DC: US Government Printing Office, 1970.
12. *Report of the Commission on the Evaluation of Pain.* SSA Pub 64-031, US Dept of Health and Human Services, Social Security Administration, Office of Disability, March 1987.
13. White EJ, Panjabi MM. *Clinical biomechanics of the spine.* Philadelphia: JB Lippincott, 1978.
14. Farfan HF. *Mechanical disorders of the low back.* Philadelphia: Lea & Febiger, 1973.
15. White AA III, Panjabi MM. *Clinical biomechanics of the spine,* 2nd ed. Philadelphia: JB Lippincott, 1990.
16. Muggleton JM, Kondracki M, Allen R. Spinal fusion for lumbar instability: does it have a scientific basis? *J Spinal Disord* 2000;13:3:200–204.
17. Ahn-H, Cho Y-W, Ahn M-W, et al. mRNA expression of cytokines and chemokines in herniated lumbar intervertebral discs. *Spine* 2002;27: 9:911–917.
18. Balkwill F. Cytokine amplification and inhibition of immune and inflammatory responses. *J Viral Hepat* 1997;4(Suppl 2):615.
19. Waddell G, Main CJ, Morris EW, et al. Chronic low back pain: psychological distress and illness behavior. *Spine* 1984;9:209
20. Inman VT, Ralston HJ, Todd F. *Human walking.* Baltimore: Williams & Wilkins, 1981.

21. Mixter WJ, Barr JS. Rupture of the intervertebral disc with involvement of the spinal canal. *N Engl J Med* 1934;211:210.
22. Eklund JA, Corlett EN. Shrinkage as a measure of the effect of load on the spine. *Spine* 1984;9:189.
23. Bernard TN Jr, Kirkaldy-Willis WH. Recognizing specific characteristics of nonspecific low back pain. *Clin Orthop* 1987;217:266–280.
24. Nachemson AL. The natural course of low back pain. *Proceedings of the American Academy of Orthopaedic Surgeons, Symposium on Idiopathic Low Back Pain,* Miami, Fl, December 1980. St. Louis: CV Mosby, 1982: 46–51.
25. Maigne R. *Diagnosis and treatment of pain of vertebral origin,* Baltimore: Williams & Wilkins, 1996.
26. Nachemson AL, Elfstrom G. Intravital dynamic pressure measurements in lumbar discs: a study of common movements, maneuvers and exercises. *Scand J Rehabil Med* 1970;1:1.
27. Forst JJ. *Contribution à l'étude de la sciatique.* Paris, Thèse no. 33, 1881.
28. Laseque EC. Quoted in De Palma A, Rothman RH. *The intervertebral disc.* Philadelphia: WB Saunders, 1970.
29. Fajersztajn J. Uber das gekreuzte schiashanomen. *Wein Klin Wochenschr* 14:41.
30. Van Akkersveeken RF. On pain patterns of patients with lumbar nerve root entrapment. *Neuro-Orthopedics* 1993;14:81.
31. Van Akkerveeken RF. On pain patterns of patients with lumbar nerve root entrapment. *Neuro-Orthopedics* 1993;14:81.
32. Hippocrates. *Librium de Affectionibus* II, 25:166.
33. Cotunnuius (Cotugno) D. *De Ischiade Nervosa. Graffer,* Vienna: 1770.
34. Wertheim-Salononson JKA. Pathologie en therapie der neuritis, myositis, zenuwgezwellen, neuralgie en myalgie. Scheltema en Holema. Amsterdam: 1911.
35. Verbiest H. Chronischer lumbaler vertebragener Schmerz: Pathomechanismus and Dianose. In: Benini A, ed. *Komplikationen and Misserfolge des lumbalen Diskus-chirurgie.* Bern: Huber, 1989.
36. Pedrini-Mille A, Weinstein JN, Found DEM, et al. Stimulation of dorsal root ganglia and degradation of rabbit annulus fibrosus. *Spine* 1990;15: 12:1252–1256.
37. Howe JF, Loeser JD, Calvin WH. Mechanosensitivity of dorsal root ganglia anal chronically injured axons: a physiological basis for the radicular pain of nerve root compression. *Pain* 1977;3:25–41.
38. Yabuki S, Igarashi T, Kikuchi S. Application of nucleus pulposus to the nerve root simultaneously reduces blood flow in dorsal root ganglion and corresponding hindpaw in the rat. *Spine* 2000;25:12:1471–1476.
39. Sarno J. *Mind over back pain.* New York: William Morrow, 1984.
40. Verbiest H. The management of cervical spondylosis. *Clin Neurosurg* 1983;20:262.
41. Zimmemann M. Regulatory functions of the nervous system; as exemplified by the spinal motor system. In: Schmidt RF. *Fundamentals of neurophysiology.* New York: Springer-Verlag, 1985:210.
42. Mooney V, Robertson J. The facet syndrome. *Clin Orthop* 1976;115: 149–156.
43. Keegan JJ, Garrett FD. The segmental distribution of the cutaneous nerves in the limbs of man. *Anat Rec* 1948;102:409.
44. Holt EP. The question of lumbar discography. *J Bone Joint Surg* 1968;50A:4:720–726.

2. THE VERTEBRAL COLUMN

The vertebral column, of which the lumbar spine is a segment, is a complex muscular ligamentous structure that supports the entire body. This structure is a neuromuscular system that is totally subservient to the nervous system, central and peripheral. The activities of the vertebral column, be they supportive or functionally kinetic, originate in the cerebral cortex, where the intended task is determined. The activity intended is ultimately submitted to the muscles of the vertebral column through the nervous pathways of the spinal cord (Fig. 2.1).

The impulses that originate in the cerebral cortex and ultimately activate the muscles occur in patterns. These patterns originally are inherent and gross but improve in accuracy, integrity, and intensity with training, practice, and performance. The specificity of the patterns is directly and instantaneously modified by a sensory feedback to the central nervous system.

Without fully understanding and implementing these patterns, normal low back function cannot be appreciated, nor can efforts to improve function and to decrease pain be instituted. This text is intended to clarify this concept and remove the current enigma.

The early studies of Wilder Penfield (1) elicited a specific muscular response on stimulation of a single neuron in the premotor cortex. He thus related specific peripheral muscular action as originating in the large Betz cells of the premotor cortex. Later studies have refuted this individual muscle response and have postulated that all movements occur as patterns (2–5). These patterns are now considered to exist in the cortex, the midbrain, the basal ganglia, and the cerebellum (6).

Just as all peripheral muscles are so activated, so are the trunk muscles of the spine, which are activated in patterns that depend on whether the intended action is to maintain stability, to initiate kinetic activity, or both (Fig. 2.2).

All motor activity occurs in two stages: planning and execution. In either stage the activation phase of the action is planned in the upper neurologic system: the cortex, midbrain, basal ganglia, and cerebellum. The details of torque and force are not considered in the cortex or midbrain, as these stages of execution are moderated in the muscular system by the spindle and Golgi systems. Numerous neurophysiologists have raised the question of whether the brain represents movement but this question remains to be answered.

The neuromuscular system supports, stabilizes, and activates the ligamentous spine, with ultimate movement occurring in the peripheral articulations (joints), which in the vertebral column are the discs and the facets. In any inappropriate movements and with unmet

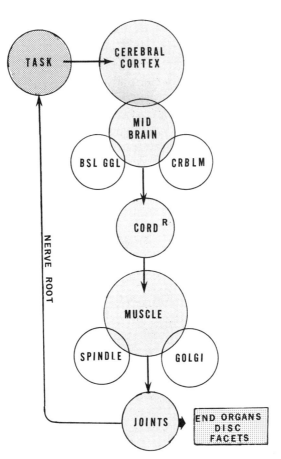

FIG. 2.1. Neurologic sequence of spinal activity. The intended movement of the individual originates in the cerebral cortex. All musculoskeletal motions occur as patterns that are ingrained in the cortex, the midbrain, basal ganglion (BSL GGL) and the cerebellum (CRBLM). From there the neurologic impulses are transmitted through the spinal cord to the extrafusal muscle fibers of the spine. The muscle contractions are moderated by the spindle system and the Golgi apparatus in relation to strength, tension, and rapidity. The muscles ultimately move the articulations points of the spine: the discs and the facets.

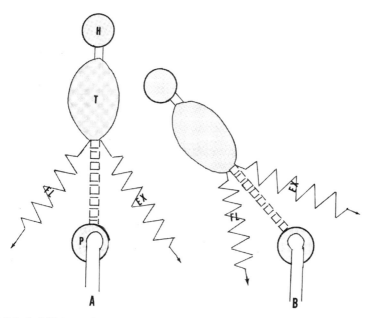

FIG. 2.2. Stabilizing and activating muscles on the vertebral column. **A:** The stable erect spine with the pelvis (P), the thorax (T), and the head (H) conforming to the center of gravity. The flexor (FL) and extensor (EX) muscles maintain its stability. **B:** Kinetic flexion with the flexors contracting isokinetically and the extensors decelerating the action.

stabilizing forces there can be resultant impairment of these distal joints resulting in pain and disability.

The neuromuscular patterns that exist in the central nervous system, once recognized, can be restored and modified by appropriate therapeutic measures (7,8,9).

THE LUMBOSACRAL SPINE

The lumbosacral spine comprises five lumbar functional units that contain these end organs: the disc and facets. Two adjacent vertebra and all their component parts comprise a *functional unit*. The *ligamentous spine* comprises the vertebra, the intervertebral discs, the longitudinal ligaments, and the facets with their capsules.

The two adjacent vertebrae within a functional unit are mechanically connected by the longitudinal ligaments, anteriorly and posteriorly, by the intervening disc annular fibers, and posteriorly by the facet joint capsules.

In the upright posture the lumbar spine structurally supports the axial compressive forces from loads of the thorax, the upper extremities, and any load the extremities may hold at a distance from the

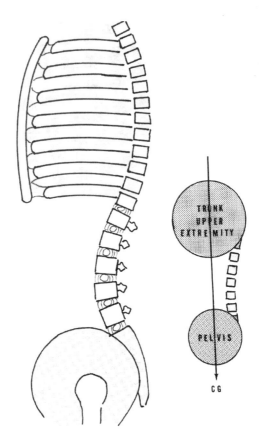

FIG. 2.3. The ligamentous spine. The lumbosacral spine basically supports two inflexible systems: the thoracic spine, which is made inflexible by the ribs, and the pelvis, which articulates between the two femoral heads. The figure to the right shows the instability of the two segments balanced by a flexible rod, the lumbar spine. CG, center of gravity.

center of gravity. The ligamentous spine is known to be unstable at loads of less than half the weight of the body, which weights in the hands augment when the arms deviate from the center of gravity (Fig. 2.3).

The mechanical support of the erect spine, being the ligamentous spine, is considered the passive subsystem, which buckles when the superimposed load, termed the *critical load of the spine,* is excessive. Initially, the external muscular system was not considered as part of the passive subsystem, but this is no longer believed to be true (10,11).

The muscular system is now considered essential for sustaining the erect spine. The extrafusal muscle fibers with their fascia and tendons form a vital portion of the stable spine (12,13). The stability of the ver-

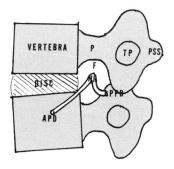

FIG. 2.4. Functional unit viewed from the side. A functional unit comprises two adjacent vertebrae separated by a disc. Posteriorly is a bony arch with the pedicles merging into the lamina, from which emerge transverse processes (TP) and join posteriorly, forming the posterior superior spine (PSS). Between the two pedicles are foramina (F) through which emerge the nerve roots (NR) that divide into the anterior primary division (APD) and the posterior primary division (PPD).

tebral column is totally dependent on co-activation of both flexor and extensor extrafusal muscle fibers in addition to the ligamentous spine (14,15).

COMPONENTS OF THE LIGAMENTOUS SPINE

The individual functional units that comprise the vertebral column contain two adjacent vertebrae separated by a hydraulic system: the intervertebral disc. These functional units afford hydraulic support against compressive forces and permit motion (Figs. 2.4 and 2.5).

THE INTERVERTEBRAL DISC

The intervertebral disc, considered one of the end organs of the neurologic sequence of spinal activity, is a hydraulic elastic structure interposed between the two adjacent vertebrae of a functional unit. A

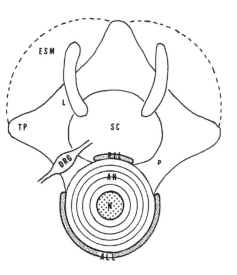

FIG. 2.5. A superior view of a lumbar vertebra. Viewed from above, a lumbar vertebra contains the following structures: the pedicles (P) emerge from the posterior–lateral aspect of the vertebral body; the transverse processes (TP), to which attach the trunk muscles (ESM); the lamina (L), from which emerge the facets (F) (zygapophyseal joints). The lamina merge posteriorly to form the spinal canal (SC), which contains the nerve roots of the cauda equina. Each root has a dorsal root ganglion (DRG). The long ligaments, anterior ligaments (ALL), and posterior ligaments (PLL) connect the vertebra and form the outer layers of the disc annulus (AN). The disc nucleus (N) is central within the annulus.

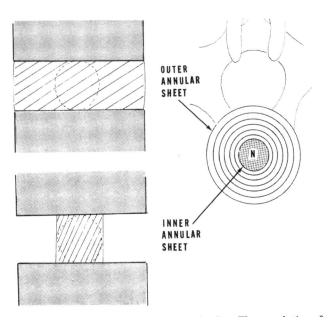

FIG. 2.6. Angular variation of collagen fibers in the disc. The angulation of the outer annular fibers is at approximately 30 degrees and is of physiologic length. The lower figure shows the annular fibers in the inner sheet near the nucleus of shorter length and more acute angle.

disc is composed of a mucopolysaccharide gel matrix that contains collagen annular fibers. These fibers, attached at opposing vertebral endplates, form sheets that cross the intervertebral space in oblique directions at approximately a 30-degree angle. The direction of the annular fibers in each sheet is completely different from that in an adjacent sheet.

The length and angulation of the annular fibers change with the change of the imposing forces on the disc (Figs. 2.6 through 2.8).

COLLAGEN FIBERS

Collagen is the building structure of all the soft tissues of the body: the ligaments, tendons, cartilage, joint capsules, skin, intervertebral disc, menisci, and so on. A collagen fiber is a complex chain of amino acids that intertwine in a trihelix with specific curvature and linkage. Eleven genetically distinct types of collagen have been assigned numbers I to XI. Each type varies in the component amino acids that form it (Fig. 2.9).

The collagen content of the disc steadily increases from the center of the nucleus to the outer annulus. The fibrous framework of the disc is built from type I and type II collagen fibrils and attains as much

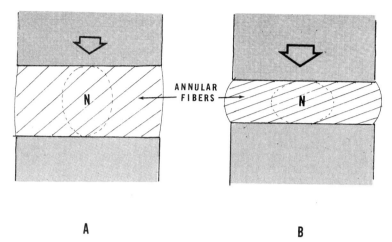

A   **B**

FIG. 2.7. Length and angle of annular fiber with compression. **A:** Relaxed disc with nucleus (N). **B:** Under compression (*arrow*) the nucleus deforms and the annular fibers change angle and length.

as 70% of the dry weight of the disc. In the disc annulus the collagen fibrils form sheets that number approximately ten to 20. The fibrils of each sheet run in the opposite direction, and judging from their angulation it is apparent that the rotational forces elongate every other lamella while relaxing the opposing lamella.

The nucleus has fewer collagen fibrils and no geometrical alignment, so their elongation is random, if at all. The hydrodynamic effect of the nucleus is from the polysaccharide matrix. The disc acts hydrodynamically to neutralize compressive forces and keep the vertebral endplates apart, which keeps the annular fibers elongated to their physiologic lengths. The hydrodynamic forces of adjacent vertebra that form a functional unit allow compression, flexion, extension, and limited rotation. Some creep is permitted within physiologic limits.

The intervertebral disc is an avascular tissue (Fig. 2.10) that receives its nutrition from imbibition. This means that for normal function during the day there must be periods of no compression, flexion–extension, rotation, or torque. Being one of the end organs of neurophysiologic function that indicate relief from compressive forces of gravity, and paraspinous muscular contraction results in inhibition.

POSTERIOR SPINAL ELEMENTS

The posterior segments of the vertebra forming the functional unit include the zygapophyseal joints (facets), the pedicles, lamina, posterior

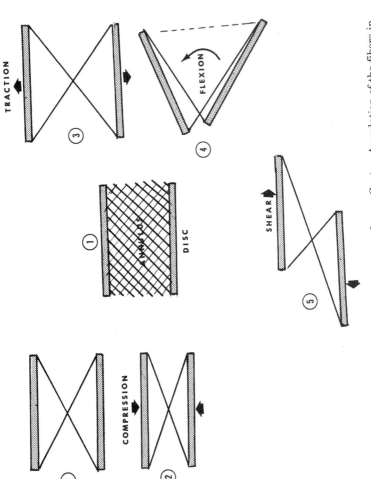

FIG. 2.8. Annular fiber angulation under various forces. Center: Angulation of the fibers in the annular sheaths: (1) uncompressed disc with its physiologic angulation of annular fibers, (2) under compression, (3) under traction forces, (4) with flexion (extension), (5) under shear forces.

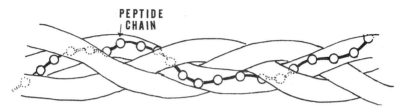

FIG. 2.9. A collagen fiber. A collagen fiber is a trihelix of amino acids in chains that intertwine. They have a physiologic curvature that uncurls when the fiber is extended and recurls when the elongating forces are eliminated. At each I intersection the chains are bonded.

superior spinous processes, the spinal canal and its contents, the foramina and its contents: the nerve roots of the cauda equina.

THE ZYGAPOPHYSEAL JOINTS: THE FACETS

The facet joints, another distal articulation in the neurologic sequence, are synovial joints. They are bony prominences arising from the lamina. They are enclosed within a synovial capsule that has sufficient redundancy to allow a large range of motion but is too thin to be a limiting tissue, although its ventral portion is reinforced by the ligamentum flavum.

At its attachment to the facets the synovium is thickened and plicated on itself. Within this plication resides small fat pads that project into the joint space by several centimeters and form a fibroadipose

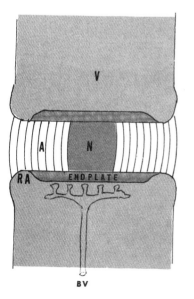

FIG. 2.10. Blood supply to the intervertebral disc. No blood vessels (BV) enter the normal disc. They approach the endplate from the bone marrow (BM) and terminate in bulbous ends. There is imbibition into the annulus (A) and nucleus (N) from compression and relaxation of the disc.

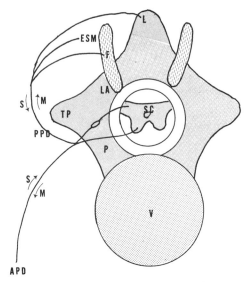

FIG. 2.11. Innervation of the facet joints. The nerve roots that emerge from the spinal cord (SC) divide immediately into the anterior primary division (APD) and posterior primary division (PPD). The latter terminates on the facets (F), the extensor spinal muscles (ESM), and the posterior ligaments (L). LA, the lamina; P, the pedicle; TP, transverse process; V, vertebra.

meniscus-like structure that performs the function of a meniscus to ensure congruency.

The facet joints are well innervated by terminal branches of the posterior primary divisions of the nerve roots after they emerge from the foramen (Fig. 2.11). They contain proprioceptive as well as nociceptive nerve endings. The facets lay in a sagittal plane, thus allowing flexion and extension of a functional unit and minimizing any lateral and rotational movement of a functional unit. As a functional unit flexes, the facets separate, as do the pedicles, and the intervertebral foramina open.

By their curved, oblique, and sagittal orientation the facets also minimize any translatory (shear) movement of adjacent vertebrae known as *listhesis*.

Clinically, the facets play a significant role in the movements of the functional unit. They prevent movement opposite to their alignment: lateral flexion and rotation. They are supplied by large proprioceptive end organs that inform the central nervous system of any movement and help coordinate that movement. They are also amply supplied by nociceptive end organs that transmit nociceptive impulses on any trauma or inflammation causing pain.

LIGAMENTS IN SPINAL FUNCTION

The ligaments of a functional unit: the anterior longitudinal, posterior longitudinal, the ligamentum flavum, the intervertebral ligaments, and the posterior supraspinatus ligaments contribute very little, if anything, to maintaining spinal stability. During the creep of two adjacent vertebrae the loss of forces in the ligaments is not considered a major factor (16,17,18).

The ligamentum flavum, which connects to the interior of the spinal canal, has significant flexibility, as it is 80% elastin and 20% collagen. It mechanically reinforces the joint capsules of the facets and prevents them from protruding into the foramen and causing compression of the nerve roots within the foramen.

The supraspinatus ligament connects the adjacent dorsal tips of the spinous processes. These ligaments contain a higher percentage of collagen fibers and show irregular alignment of the fibers, thus allowing only limited movement of the posterior elements of the units.

The interspinous ligaments connect adjacent transverse processes and are divided into three portions: ventral, middle, and dorsal. These ligaments contain more collagen than elastin and thus have less elasticity and elongation. Their function is to limit passive and active range of motion of each functional unit. They are avascular and poorly innervated, so their role as proprioceptors or nociceptors remains uncertain.

The posterior and anterior longitudinal ligaments play a more specific role in spinal function. They run longitudinally along adjacent vertebra and are connected to the vertebral bodies. At the intervertebral spaces occupied by the discs they literally form the outer annular portions of the discs. They are amply innervated by nociceptive nervous end organs. The posterior longitudinal ligament is considered prominent in transmitting pain when inflamed from a damaged disc.

MUSCULAR SYSTEM OF THE LOW BACK

The muscles of the low back, the lumbosacral spine, were initially considered to act with linear force, with their action involving direct distances from origin and insertion. They now are understood to be multisegmental and to act on a given segment in various directions from various points of attachment. In this manner they act around various axes of rotation.

Different tasks require different sequences of motion acting between isometric and isotonic activities. Energy costs in the performance of a specific action are important, as this relates to a waste of energy in ineffectual neuromuscular function.

The passive subsystem that maintains the static erect spine includes the fascia of muscles as well as the disc fibers, ligaments, and joint capsules. All extrafusal muscle fibers are enclosed within a fascial sheath that elongates as the muscle elongates and passively shortens as the muscle contracts.

The thoracolumbar fascia encloses all the erector spinae and quadratus lumborum muscles. The thoracolumbar fascia by its attachments stabilizes the erect spine and mechanically reextends the spine. The spine flexes laterally and assists in trunk rotation.

The erect spine is made stable by virtue of these fascial sheaths, which are made taut when the back muscles contract along with the deep oblique abdominal muscles, the transversus abdominis and the latissimus dorsi, whose posterior insertions create the intracompartment of the erector muscles.

The transversus muscles are the activators of the anterior compartment (the abdominal air bag) and with the latissimus dorsi are the activators of the erector spinae compartment. The other abdominal muscles—the obliques and the rectus abdominis—are essentially flexors and rotators but not stabilizers.

In any upper-extremity action there is contraction of the transversus muscles in anticipation of the pending action with trunk stabilization. This action is termed *feed-forward,* as compared with *feedback* from a completed action.

Four major extrafusal muscles of the trunk furnish the stability of the trunk and functions in the kinetic action in the thorax with upper-extremity activities. These trunk muscles are the external oblique (Fig. 2.12), the anterior oblique abdominal (Fig. 2.13), and the transversus abdominis muscles (Fig. 2.14). The quadratus lumborum muscles are the extensor trunk muscles that coordinate in the tubular stability of the trunk (Fig. 2.15).

This subsystem of spinal stability, with the fascia forming the tubular structures, remains under control of sufficient isometric contraction of the trunk muscles. The transversus abdominis and the quadratus lumborum muscles are essential for spinal stability, and the other abdominal flexor muscles are kinetic muscles that move the trunk in flexion, lateral flexion, and rotation along with upper-extremity activity. They should remain "quiet" when only stability is required.

In any upper-extremity action, such as lifting, pushing, and pulling, the trunk must become stable. It does this by contraction of the transversus abdominis muscles.

Certain occupational activities impose cyclic or prolonged trunk flexion postures that cause low back disorders. These cyclic or prolonged postures have caused "creeping" of adjacent vertebrae: the superior on the inferior.

This creep cannot be attributed to ligamentous laxity or to facet capsular laxity, so studies imply that it is related to disc narrowing that

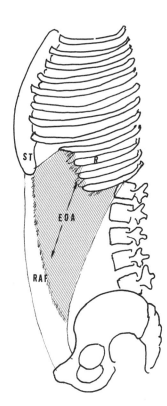

FIG. 2.12. External oblique abdominal muscles. The external oblique abdominal muscles (EOA) originate from the lateral inferior surfaces of the ninth to twelfth rib (R) and the sternum (ST). It inserts on the anterior half of the iliac crest and the fascia of the rectus abdominis muscles (RAF). This muscle flexes the spine forward and sideways.

causes the instability. The fluid contents of the disc change over a routine 24-hour period because of compressive forces (19–23). These compressive changes are accentuated in the cyclic and prolonged flexed postures, and the disc narrows, causing instability as the ligaments and annular fibers are no longer under the same tension.

The musculature, which is the major stabilizing force, is also destabilized in this creeping action because of loss of the ligamentous–muscular reflex. This reflex is initiated by the mechanoreceptors in ligaments, the facet capsules, and even the annular fibers that activate the muscles of that joint.

The mechanoreceptors of the spinal ligaments, disc, and joint capsule elicit reflex activity in the multifidus muscles of the spine (23,24), which is one of the stabilizing erector spinae muscles. Fatigue of the muscles in cyclic and prolonged flexion may diminish the protective muscle reflex and allow creep, with resultant instability by reduction of protective reflex from mechanoreceptor desensitization caused by laxity in the viscoelastic tissues of the spine: the ligaments and annular fibers (Fig. 2.16) (25,26).

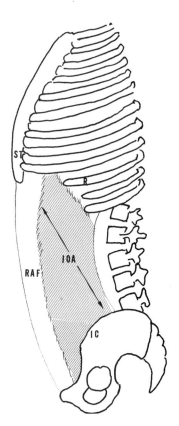

FIG. 2.13. Internal oblique abdominal muscles. The internal oblique abdominal muscles (IOA) originate from the lateral two-thirds of the inguinal ligament and the anterior one-third of the iliac crest (IC) and insert on the pubis and the linea alba of the fascia of the rectus abdominis muscles (RAF). Their action is to flex and rotate the trunk on the pelvis.

A 50-minute period of cyclic or prolonged flexion of the spine causes an 85% reduction of the muscular stabilizing forces of the spine that begins in the first 5 minutes. A 10-minute rest period has been shown to be too short to restore the reflex-stabilizing effects of the musculature to a functional level.

This finding is a frequently ignored ergonomic factor in preventing low back disorders in which persons performing activities demanding cyclic flexion or prolonged flexed positions do not get rest periods of sufficient length and frequency to restore the sensitivity of the mechanoreceptors and the protective muscular reflex.

As the type of muscular contraction is predominant in well-coordinated spinal function, the various types of contraction merit consideration:

1. *Concentric:* Contraction that produces motion through its shortening. The internal force of the muscle exceeds the external force of resistance.

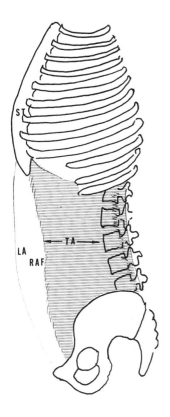

FIG. 2.14. Transversus abdominis muscles. The transversus abdominis muscles (TA) is the deepest abdominal muscle. It originates from the lateral one-third of the inguinal ligament, the anterior two-thirds of the iliac crest (IC), the inner edges of the lower six-rib costal cartilages, and the sternum (ST). It inserts on the linea alba (LA) and the fascia of the rectus abdominis muscles (RAF). Its action is to constrict the abdominal contents and enforce the tubular abdominal cavity. By contraction of the transversus abdominis muscles the air bag is created by simultaneous contraction of the diaphragm and the pelvic muscles.

2. *Eccentric:* This contraction develops tension within the muscle as it shortens. Deceleration is an example of eccentric contraction.
3. *Isometric:* A contraction in which there is no external movement as the muscle does not shorten but does develop tension.
4. *Isotonic:* Contraction occurs when internal contraction and external force are equal and no movement occurs.
5. *Anisotonic:* Contraction occurs during motion and is either concentric (positive work) or eccentric (negative work).

The intrafusal nerve supply (spindle and Golgi systems) moderates the extrafusal muscles because the torque and strength of a muscular contraction are not determined at higher levels (Fig. 2.17).

THE STATIC SPINE

The erect spine consists of four physiologic curves: the lumbar and cervical lordosis and the thoracic and sacral kyphosis. All four conform to the center of gravity (Fig. 2.18).

The lumbosacral curve, of clinical pertinence in this text, has routinely been measured at the Cobb angle (Fig. 2.19). The curvature is

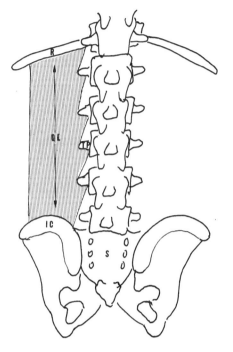

FIG. 2.15. Quadratus lumborum muscles. The quadratus lumborum muscles (QL) originate from the ilio-lumbar ligament and the posterior part of the iliac crest (IC). It inserts on the inferior border of the last rib (R) and the transverse processes (TP) of the upper four lumbar vertebrae. Its action is lateral flexion of the lumbar vertebrae, and by its attachments to the erector spinae fascia act as stabilizers.

made by drawing lines parallel to the inferior surface of the twelfth vertebra (T12). This curve postulates that each segment has identical angulations and curve and that the total curve (lordosis) is represented (Fig. 2.19).

This was questioned by Harrison et al. (27,28), who measured the total lordotic curve as a total of each relative rotational angle (RRA). The RRAs are measured from vertical lines drawn from the posterior surface of each vertebra and are measured at each segment, giving a more physiologic lordotic curvature and stating the specific functional unit curvature (Fig. 2.20).

STABILITY OF THE STATIC SPINE

The erect spine and the spine during any physical activity remain stable by the extrafusal muscles of the trunk and their fascia as a result of "tubular" structures. The tendons and the fascia of the muscles of the trunk and the latissimus dorsi muscle combine at the raphe, sending sheaths that encircle the extensor muscles: the quadratus lumborum and the erector spinae muscles. The compartments formed are located posteriorly and, with the anterior compartment of the abdominal cavity, afford stability of the vertebral column (Figs. 2.21–2.24).

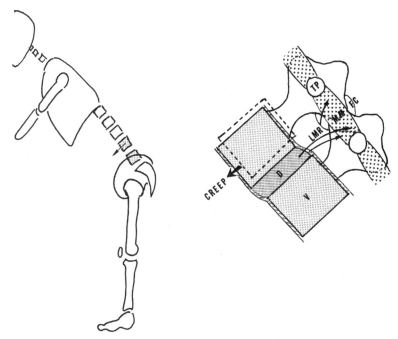

FIG. 2.16. Protective ligamentous–muscular reflex. The left figure depicts the cyclic or prolonged flexed posture of many occupations. The right figure shows "creep" of the superior vertebra on the lower adjacent vertebra (V) with narrowing of the disc space (D). The neurologic reflex (LMR) from the longitudinal ligament, the disc annular fibers, and the facet capsule (FC) innervates the multifidus muscle (MM), which attaches to the transverse processes (TP). See the text for details.

Stability of the spine has been proposed as occurring from contraction of the deep vertebral muscles: the intersegmental intertransversalis and interspinalis, the lumbar multifidus, longissimus thoracis pars lumborum, and the medial fibers of the quadratus lumborum (Figs. 2.25 and 2.26).

These muscles are primarily extensors of the low back when they contract bilaterally but are lateral flexors and rotators when they contract unilaterally.

These small muscles are considered spinal segmental stabilizers of the lumbar spine (29). The other trunk muscles, the external oblique and internal oblique, are global muscles in that they activate the spine while the small intrinsic muscles stabilize the spine. Weakness or failure of these small muscles to contract has been found to cause functional impairment of the low back. All these muscles are vital in the proposed neurologic sequence of low back function (26,29).

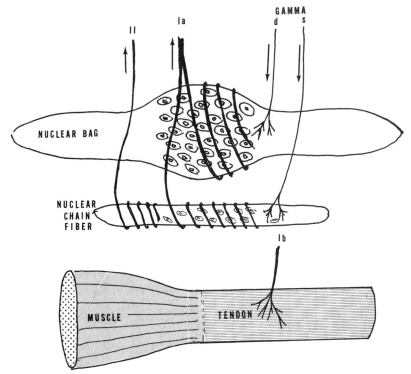

FIG. 2.17. Spindle and Golgi systems of muscular control. The upper drawing shows a nuclear bag and chain fiber encircled by sensory nerves (Ia and II). These are afferent nerves to the cord transmitting information to the cord as to length (via spindle) and force (via Golgi). The spindle system is constantly "reset" by motor efferent fibers. The Golgi apparatus is within the muscle tendinous system with afferent nerve fibers to the cord via Ib (bottom figure).

THE KINETIC LUMBAR SPINE AND THE LUMBAR-PELVIC RHYTHM

The kinetic spine functions in a well-coordinated pattern known as the *lumbar pelvic rhythm* (Fig. 2.27).

Most bending (flexing) and lifting activities are three-dimensional in that they combine forward flexion, lateral flexion, and rotation (Fig. 2.28) (28–30). Flexion occurs by contraction of the superficial oblique abdominal flexors and the rectus femoris. These flexors contract with appropriate force and speed according to the intended task. In the early phase of flexion the extensors (antagonists) contract eccentrically.

During the later part of trunk flexion the extensors relax with a diminution of myoelectric activity, as the studies of Floyd and Silver showed (31). This diminution of the antagonist contraction they

(text continues on page 46)

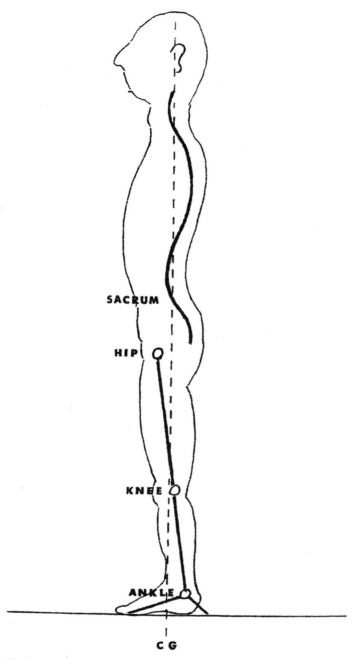

FIG. 2.18. Posture: relationship to center of gravity. The four curves of the spine (*dark curved line*) all relate to the center of gravity (CG).

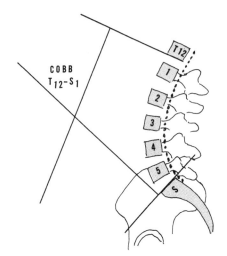

FIG. 2.19. Cobb angle of lordosis. The Cobb measurement of lumbar lordosis is shown.

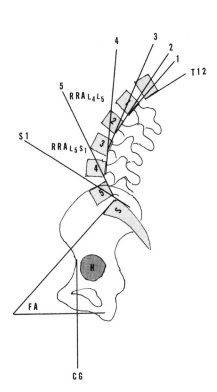

FIG. 2.20. Elliptical modeling of the normal sagittal lumbar curvature. Relative rotational angles are drawn from vertical lines drawn from each vertebral posterior surface. The RRA L5–S1 and RRA L4–L5 indicate the degree of curvature at these levels showing greater curvature at these two levels as compared with other levels. FA, Ferguson angle. (Modified from Janik TJ, Harrison DD, Cailliet R, et al. Elliptical modeling of the normal sagittal lumbar curvature. *J Spinal Disord* 1998;5:430–439.)

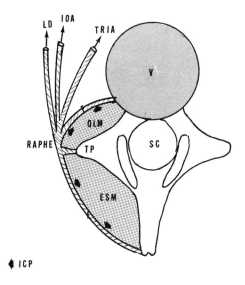

FIG. 2.21. Intracompartmental pressures. The latissimus dorsi muscle (LD), the internal oblique abdominal (IOA), and the transversus internal abdominal muscle (TRIA) merge at the raphe and send fascial sheaths (F) that encircle the quadratus lumborum muscle (QLM) and connect to the transverse process (TP) of the vertebrae. A posterior sheath surrounds the erector spinae muscles (ESM). The compartment formed acts as a tubular structure that stabilizes the spinal column.

THE "AIR BAG" THEORY

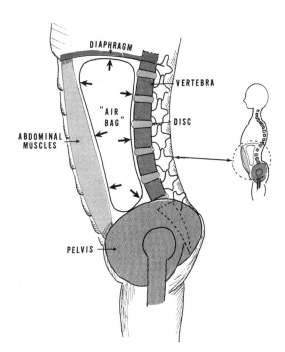

FIG. 2.22. Abdominal air bag concept. The air bag concept of support of the spine is based on a "bag" within the abdominal cavity with the diaphragm placed superiorly; the pelvis, inferiorly; the abdominal muscles, anteriorly; and the spine, posteriorly.

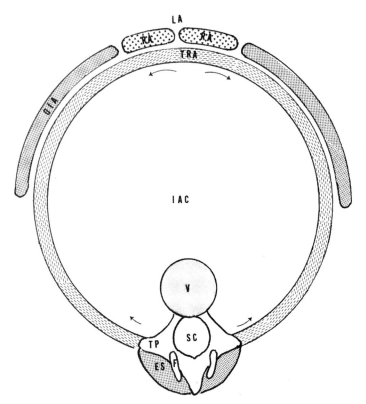

FIG. 2.23. Components of the air bag. The abdominal cavity is totally surrounded by the transversus abdominis muscles (TRA) whose horizontal fibers attach posteriorly to the fascia of the compartment containing the quadratus lumborum and erector spinae (ES) muscles. The more superficial abdominal muscles are the internal oblique (OIA), whose fibers run obliquely, and the rectus abdominis (RA) muscles, whose fibers run vertically and fuse anteriorly at the linea alba (LA). The OIA muscles rotate the trunk and the RA muscles flex the trunk. V, the vertebrae; F, the facets; TP, the transverse processes; and SC, the spinal canal.

termed *flexion relaxation* and implied it was reflex activity from impulses generated from the stretched ligaments of the posterior elements of the spine and from receptors in the facet (zygapophyseal) capsules that are stretched at the end of flexion.

These proprioceptors apparently decrease the rapidity of flexion by activating the deep muscles, the multifidus, the quadratus lumborum, and the iliocostalis, which become silent, although they continue to exhibit tone.

PREPARATORY TRUNK MOTIONS
Before there is any kinetic action of the body, attention must be given to insure adequate preparatory motions. Any upper extremity invoked

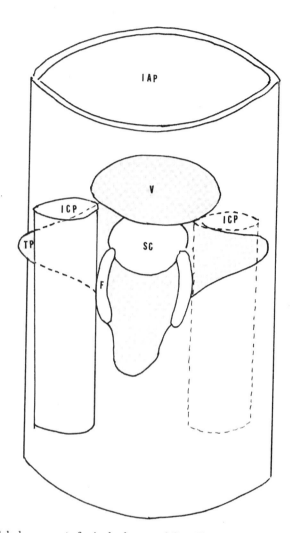

FIG. 2.24. Tubular concept of spinal column stability. The spine is supported by three tubular structures: (IAP) Intraabdominal pressure, (ICP) intracompartmental pressure and the spinous structure of adjacent functional units. Each unit consists of two adjacent vertebrae (V), facets (F), transverse processes (TP) and a spinal canal (SC). These "tubular" structures support the erect spine and add stability when there is added upper-extremity activity that flex, extend, and/or rotate the spine.

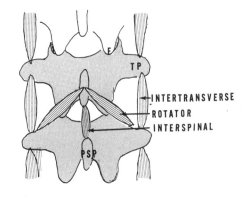

FIG. 2.25. Intersegmental muscles. The small vertebral muscles are the intertransversalis and interspinales, which connect the transverse processes and spinous processes of two adjoining vertebrae. They have segmental nerve supply but are too small to have any significant torque capability. They are probably proprioceptive in their function. TP, transverse processes; PSP, posterior spinous process.

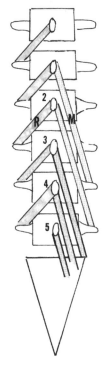

FIG. 2.26. Lumbar multifidus muscles. The multifidus muscles are the most medial of the lumbar muscles and connect vertebra to vertebra. They have five bands that connect spinous processes together and that connect the adjacent lamina between the lumbar vertebrae and the sacrum.

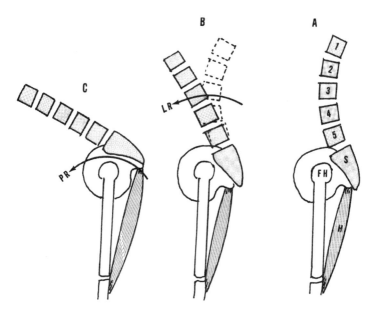

FIG. 2.27. Lumbar pelvic rhythm. (A) The erect static spine with physiological lordosis and the pelvis in the neutral position. The hamstring muscles (H) contract isometrically stabilizing the pelvis. (B) Beginning trunk flexion, with no pelvic rotation, the lordosis becomes a kyphosis as the lumbar spine rotates (LR). (C): When lumbar kyphosis is reached the pelvis has also undergone full rotation (PR). The lumbar spine and pelvis rotate in a rhythm.

in any activity perturbs the balance of the entire body, the body mass, as it relates to the center of gravity (32,33,34).

It has been postulated that before any significant activity that displaces the body mass a feed-forward reflex occurs. This activity of the central nervous system instantly alerts and prepares the total body mass for the impending action. This activates the muscles of the trunk to minimize the postural disturbance caused by the upper extremity and any weights held away from the body (35,36). This action has been termed *feed-forward,* as compared with the term *feedback,* which involves informing the central nervous system that the intended action has been accomplished (37–48).

As an upper extremity moves away from the center of gravity the trunk muscles react with a tonic (isometric) contraction. In forward arm movement there is no preactivation (according to electromyographic studies) of the transverse abdominal muscles to increase the intraabdominal pressure (IAP) (49–53) so merely stabilization results and not any feed-forward activity.

As the arm(s) moves forward, the body instantly and appropriately leans backward to remain over the center of gravity (Figs. 2.29 and 2.30).

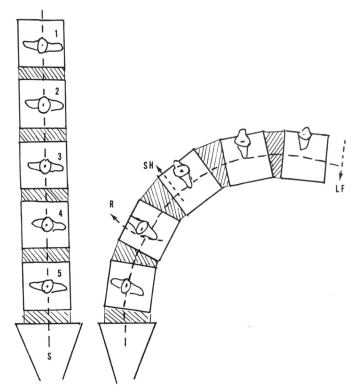

FIG. 2.28. Three-dimensional flexion. The erect spine is shown on the left, and flexion is shown on the right, which shows that as the spine flexes, it flexes laterally and simultaneously rotates when movement is slightly off center.

The increase in the intraabdominal pressure from the transversus abdominis muscles apparently also produces some trunk extension by exerting a force between the diaphragm and the pelvic floor, but these changes are minimal.

The superficial abdominal flexors contract sufficiently to shift the body mass ahead of the CE (36–38). The opposite would occur were the arm extended backward over the CE.

Currently, there is debate about whether the shift from the center of gravity of the body mass is controlled by the feed-forward activation of the trunk muscles (45,46) or whether the shift relates to the position of the hip joint and its muscles with the trunk following (47,48). The answer is yet to be found but there is muscular activity of all the trunk muscles as well as the muscles of the hip joint (49–55).

In viewing the proposed neurologic sequence of spinal activity (Fig. 2.1), it becomes apparent that a complex muscular system must

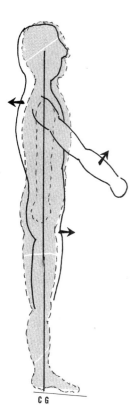

FIG. 2.29. Feed-forward motion. The erect upper body (*dotted lines*) in its relationship to the center of gravity (CG) moves backward (*horizontal arrow*) as the arm(s) move forward. The pelvis also moves forward slightly, increasing the lumbar lordosis.

be addressed to understand ultimate damage to the articulations, the discs and the facets, that present symptoms and findings to the clinician examining and treating the low back impairments (53–55).

Radiculopathy

Pain referred from the low back, described as sciatica by Forst (56) and later by Laseque (57), is termed *radiculopathy:* pain transmitted intrasegmentally by a spinal nerve (58). The nerve root in its passage through the intervertebral foramen may be painful because of inflammation of the sensory nerve fibers and/or its dura within the foramen (Fig. 2.31) or the sensory fibers of the motor root. The motor roots, initially considered efferent and strictly motor, are now considered to be mixed with afferent sensory fibers.

Transmitted pain when a peripheral nerve or its dorsal root ganglion is inflamed may undergo two main types of nerve root degeneration: axonal degeneration or segmental demyelination (59). In axonal degeneration the axon death leads to secondary breakdown of the myelin sheath, termed *Wallerian degeneration.* In segmental demyeli-

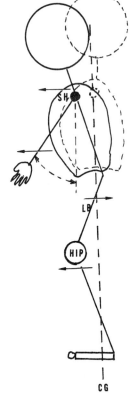

FIG. 2.30. Preparatory trunk muscle activity. The body mass (*dotted*) shows the dependent arms at the side. As the arm(s) move forward (*curved arrow*) at the shoulder joint (SH), the upper body mass (thorax and head) moves forward ahead of the center of gravity (CG). The low back (LB) extensors become activated and the hips move forward.

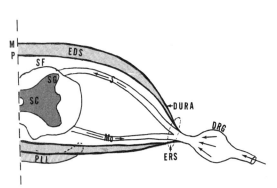

FIG. 2.31. The nerve root. The nerve root and its fibers: (S) sensory afferent and (MO) motor efferents are contained within a dural sheath that contains spinal fluid (SF). DRG, dorsal root ganglion; EDS, the epidural space; ERS, the external root space; PLL, posterior longitudinal ligament; SC, the spinal cord with its two layers: M, meningeal and P, proximal; SG, substantia gelatinosa.

nation the Schwann cells and myelin sheath are damaged but the axon remains basically intact. In most traumas both types of degeneration occur to a varying degree from transient neuropraxia to axonotmesis. [Taber's *Cyclopedic Medical Dictionary* defines *neuropraxia* as "the condition in which, due to trauma, a nerve no longer conducts even though its anatomic continuity is not interrupted." It defines *axonotmesis* as "nerve injury that damages the nerve tissue without actually severing the nerve" (60).]

Retrograde degeneration may occur to involve the nerve cell. Sunderland (61) defined five different degrees of injury. In his first degree he described a loss of conductivity of the axis cylinders without any gross apparent break in the continuity of the structure with good expected regeneration. By grade IV there is damage of the axon and perineurium but the nerve remains grossly intact, although regeneration is poor. With these stages it becomes apparent that intervention in the early stage is mandatory to prevent further degeneration (58).

According to Gunn (58) there are characteristic changes in the receptor muscle (of the myotome nerve supply) and its peripheral receptors. In the normal muscle the receptor site of the motor nerve is very specific and localized with the released acetylcholine stimulating the motor endplate (62). After denervation the sensitive area spreads along the surface membrane of the entire muscle fiber, resulting in supersensitivity (63,64).

A segmental nerve is a mixed nerve carrying both afferent and efferent fibers: sensory, motor, and autonomic. Nerve impairment can affect any or all of these components, and according to Gunn occurs in prespondylosis at the foraminal level.

These dysfunctions are autonomic, affecting the smooth muscles of the blood vessels, the piloerector muscles, and the sweat glands. The motor nerve supply interested Gunn the most. He believes that compression recurring at the foraminal levels as spondylosis progresses during gradual disc degeneration causes mild nerve degeneration with muscle segmental contraction that results in muscle shortening: limited range of motion, nodularity, and even muscle pain and sensitivity (Fig. 2.32).

With progressive neuropathy there are reflex changes, loss of muscle strength, and dermatomal degrees of loss of sensation. In early degeneration the impulses proceed to allow normal muscle contraction and no loss of sensation, but the isolated muscle fibers contract as their sensitivity to acetylcholine increases. Hence, clinically, muscle nodules are palpable in the myotomal regions of the affected nerve root impingement when an acute injury occurs. Reflexes, muscle strength, and dermatomal impairment are not clinically discernible.

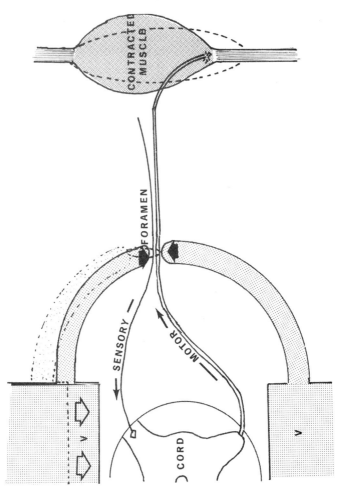

FIG. 2.32. Neuropathy from foraminal stenosis. The foramen that narrows (*dark arrows*) from disc degeneration bringing the vertebrae (V) closer together (*open arrows*) compresses the nerve roots, irritating the muscle fibers that cause sustained contraction of the muscle fibers.

REFERENCES

1. Penfield W, Rasmussen T. *The cerebral cortex of man: a clinical study of the localization of function.* New York: Macmillan, 1950.
2. Kakei S, Hoffman DS, Strick PL. Muscle and movement representation in the primary motor cortex. *Science* 1999;285:2136–2139.
3. Shumway-Cook A, Woollacott M. *Motor control: theory and practical application.* Baltimore: Williams & Wilkins, 1995.
4. Baringa M. Remapping the motor cortex. *Science* 1995;268:1696–1698
5. Schoot GD. Penfield's homunculus: a note on cerebral cartography. *J Neurol Neurosurg Psychiatry* 1993;56:329–333.

6. Raymond JL, Lisberger SG, Mauk MD. The cerebellum: a neuronal learning machine. *Science* 1996;272:1126–1131.
7. Bernstein N. *The co-ordination and regulation of movements.* New York: Pergamon Press, 1967.
8. Denier van der Gon JJ, Coolen ACC, Erkelens CJ, et al. Self-organizing neural mechanisms possibly responsible for muscle coordination. In: Winters J, Woo SL-O, eds. *Multiple muscle systems: biomechanics and movement organization.* New York: Springer-Verlag, 1990:335–342.
9. Pearcy M. A personal communication, Oxford England, 1980. Quoted in Farfan HF. Form and function of the musculoskeletal system as revealed by mathematical analysis of the lumbar spine. *Spine* 1995;2:1462–1474.
10. Bogduk N, Macintosh JE, Pearcy MJ. A universal model of the lumbar back muscles in the upright position. *Spine* 1992;17:897.
11. Macintosh JE, Bogduk N, Pearcy MJ. The effects of flexion on the geometry and actions of the lumbar erector spinae. *Spine* 1993;18:884.
12. Crisco JJ, Panjabi MM. Postural biomechanical stability and gross muscular architecture of the spine. In: Winters J, Woo SL-O, eds. *Multiple muscle systems: biomechanics and movement organization.* New York: Springer-Verlag, 1990:438–450.
13. Pennisi E. Tilting against a major theory of movement control. *Science* 1996;272:32–33.
14. Panjabi MM. The stabilizing system of the spine. Part 1: function, dysfunction, adaptation and enhancement. *J Spinal Disord* 1992;5:383.
15. Panjabi MM. The stabilizing system of the spine. Part 2: neutral zone and instability hypothesis. *J Spinal Disord* 1992;5:390–396.
16. Eyre DR. Collagens of the disc. In: Ghosh P, ed. *The biology of the intervertebral disc,* vol 1. Boca Raton, Fl: CRC Press, 1988.
17. Tillman LJ, Cummins GS. Biological mechanisms of connective tissue mutability. In: Cummins DP, Nelson RM, eds. *Dynamics of human biological tissues.* Philadelphia: FA Davis, 1992:1–44.
18. Solomonow M, Bing-He Zhou EE, Baratta RV, et al. Biomechanics of increased exposure to lumbar injury caused by cyclic loading. Part 1: Loss of reflexive muscular stabilization. *Spine* 1999;24:2426–2434.
19. Adams M, Dolan P, Hutton W. Diurnal variations in the stresses on the lumbar spine. *Spine* 1987;12:130–137.
20. Botsford D, Esses S, Ogilvie-Harris D. In vivo diurnal variations in intervertebral disc volume and morphology. *Spine* 1994:19:935–940.
21. Dolan P, Benjamin E, Adams M. Diurnal changes in bending and compressive stresses acting on the lumbar spine. *J Bone Joint Surg (Br)* 1993:75(Suppl):22.
22. Dunlap R, Adams M, Hutton W. Disc space narrowing and the lumbar facet joint. *J Bone Joint Surg (Br)* 1984:66:706–710.
23. Eklund J, Corlettt E. Shrinkage as a measure of the effect of load on the spine. *Spine* 1984:9:189–194.
24. Indahl A, Kaigle A, Reikeras O, et al. Interaction between porcine lumbar intervertebral disc, zygapophyseal joints, and paraspinous muscles. *Spine* 1997:22:2834–2840.
25. Stubbs M, Harris M, Solomonow M, et al. Ligamentous-muscular protective reflex in the lumbar spine of the feline. *J Electromyogr Kinesiol* 1998:8:197–204.
26. Potvin JR, O'Brien PR. Trunk muscle co-contraction increases during fatiguing, isometric, lateral bend exertions. *Spine* 1998:23:774–780.

27. Harrison DE, Harrison DD, Cailliet R, Janik TJ, Holland B. Radiographic Analysis of Lumbar Lordosis: Centroid, Cobb, TRALL, Harrison Posterior Tangent Methods. *Spine* 2001;26:235–242.
28. Janik TJ, Harrison DD, Cailliet R, Troyanovich SJ, Harrison DE. Can the agittal lumbar curvature be closely approximated by and ellipse? *J Orthopedic Res* 1998;6:766–770.
29. McGill SM. A myoelectrically based dynamic three-dimensional model to predict loads on lumbar spine tissues during lateral bending. *J Biomech* 1992;25:395–414.
30. Thelen DG, Schultz AB, Ashton-Miller JA. Co-contraction of lumbar muscles during development of time-varying tri-axial moments. *J Orthop Res* 1995;13:390–398.
31. Floyd WF, Silver PHS. Function of the erector spinae muscles in flexion of the trunk. *Lancet* 1951;133–143.
32. Bouisset S, Zattara M. A sequence of postural adjustments precedes voluntary movement. *Neurosci Lett* 1981;22:263–270.
33. Horak FB, Esselman P, Anderson ME, et al. The effects of movement velocity, mass displaced, and task certainty on associated postural adjustments made by normal and hemiplegic individuals. *J Neurol Neurosurg Psychiatry* 1984;47:1020–1028.
34. Aruin As, Latash ML. Directional specificity of postural muscles in feedforward postural reactions during fast voluntary arm movements. *Exp Brain Res* 1995;103:323–332.
35. Friedle WG, Hallet M, Simon SR. Postural adjustments associated with rapid voluntary arm movements. II Biomechanical analysis. *J Neurol Neurosurg Psychiatry* 1988;51:232–243.
36. Hodges PW, Richardson CA. Relationship between limb movement speed and associated contraction of the trunk muscles. *Ergonomics* 1997; 40:1220–1230.
37. Hodges PW, Gandevia SC, Richardson CA. Contractions of specific abdominal muscles in postural tasks are affected by respiratory maneuvers. American Physiological Society 1997.
38. Hodges P, Cresswell A, Thorstensson A. Preparatory trunk motion accompanies rapid upper limb movement. *Exp Brain Res* 1990;124:69–79.
39. Belenkii V, Gurfinkel VS, Paltsev Y. Elements of control of voluntary movements. *Biofizika* 1967;12:135–141.
40. Tyler AE, Hasan Z. Qualitative discrepancies between trunk muscle activity and dynamic postural requirements at the initiation of reaching movements performed while sitting. *Exp Brain Res* 1995;107:87–95.
41. Eng JJ, Winter DA, MacKinnon CD, et al. Interaction of the reactive moments and centre of mass displacement for postural control during voluntary arm movements. *Neurosci Res Commun* 1992;11:73–80.
42. Massion J, Popov K, Fabre JC, et al. Is the erect posture in microgravity based on the control of trunk orientation or center of mass position. *Exp Brain Res* 1997;114:384–389.
43. Hayes KC. Biomechanics of postural control. *Exerc Sport Sci Rev* 1982; 10:363–391.
44. Cresswell AG, Oddsson L, Thorstensson A. The influence of sudden perturbations on trunk muscle activity and intraabdominal pressure while standing. *Exp Brain Res* 1994;98:336–341.
45. Bartelink DL. The role of intra-abdominal pressure in relieving the pressure on the lumbar vertebral discs. *J Bone Joint Surg (Br)* 1957;39: 718–725.

46. Daggfeldt K, Thorstensson A. The role of intra-abdominal pressure in spinal unloading. *J Biomech* 1998;30:1149–1155.
47. Grillner S, Nilsson J, Thorstensson A. Intra-abdominal pressure changes during natural movements in man. *Acta Physiol Scand* 1978; 103:275–283.
48. O'Sullivan PB, Twomey L, Allison GT. Altered abdominal muscle recruitment in patients with chronic back pain following a specific exercise intervention. *JOSPT* 1998;27:114–124.
49. Hodges PW. Is there a role for transversus abdominis in lumbopelvic stability? *Man Ther* 1999;4:74–86.
50. Hodges PW, Richardson CAA. Transversus abdominis and the superficial abdominal muscles are controlled independently in a postural task. *Neurosci Lett* 1999;265:91–94.
51. Hodges PW, Richardson CA. Delayed postural contraction of transversus abdominis in low back pain associated with movement of the lower limb. *J Spinal Disord*1998;11:46–56.
52. Morgan FP, King T. Primary instability of lumbar vertebrae as a common cause of low back pain. *J Bone Joint Surg* 1957;39B:622.
53. Hodges PW, Richardson CA. Inefficient muscular stabilization of the lumbar spine associated with low back pain. *Spine* 1996;21:2640–2650.
54. Cholewicki J, McGill SM. Mechanical stability of the in vivo lumbar spine: implications for injury and chronic low back pain. *Clin Biomech* 1996;11:1–15.
55. Hodges PW, Richardson CA. Delayed postural contraction of transversus abdominis in low back pain associated with movement of the lower limb. *J Spinal Disord* 199811:46–56.
56. Forst JJ. Contribution à l'étude clinique de la sciatique. Paris. Thèse, No. 33, 1881.
57. Laseque CH. Consideration sur la sciatique. *Arch Gen Med* 1864;2 (Serie 6,Tome 4):558–580.
58. Gunn CC, Milbrandt WE. Early and subtle signs in low back sprain. *Spine* 1978;3:100–114.
59. Thomas CL, ed. *Taber's cyclopedic medical dictionary,* 6th ed. Philadelphia: FA Davis, 1989.
60. Howe JF, Loeser JD, Calvin WH. Mechanosensitivity of dorsal root ganglia and chronically injured axons: a physiological basis for the radicular pain of nerve root compression. *Pain* 1977;3:25–41.
61. Sunderland S. Classification of peripheral nerve injuries producing loss of function. *Brain* 1952;74:491–516.
62. Del Costillo J, Katz B. On the localization of acetylcholine receptors. *J Physiol* 1955;128:159.
63. Cannon WB, Rosenblueth A. *The supersensitivity of denervated structures.* New York: Macmillan, 1949:122, 185.
64. Rosenblueth A, Luco V. A study of denervated mammalian skeletal muscle. *Am J Physiol* 1937;120:781–797.

3. THE INTERVERTEBRAL DISC

In evaluating the patient (Chapter 1) the disc has been termed the *bête noire* of low back disorders. The disc is the major joint activated in the neurologic sequence of the vertebral column function (Fig. 2.1). It is veritably at the core of spinal function and when it is damaged by faulty body function becomes the site of impairment and the basis of resultant pain.

The term *discogenic disease* has emerged so frequently in the medical literature that it is now supposed that there is such a disease. Where there is a "disease" it emanates from a damaged, not a diseased, disc. It is the anatomic site of impairment and pain, and involves the functional spine. Therefore it merits all the attention paid to it: its structure, function, and role in pathology.

The original vertebral column in embryonic development is a continuous, unsegmented condensation of mesenchyme around the notochord and is surrounded at regular intervals by small, paired branches of the primary aorta. The first sign of segmentation in the column is a differentiation into alternate light and dark bands. The light bands ultimately form into vertebral bodies at each level of aortic branch arteries. The dark bands become the intervertebral discs (1,2) (Fig. 3.1).

The light bands grow rapidly and differentiate into cartilage. The embryonic dark bands grow more slowly, and their peripheral cells differentiate into fibroblasts that align themselves in an outward convex lamellar pattern and soon form collagen (3). Primary centers of ossification appear in the cartilage of the vertebral bodies, and the cells in the primitive disc develop a "mucoid break" that gradually disappears.

The annulus fibrosus is built up of fibroblasts in concentric lamellae of fibrous tissue and fibrocartilage. Histologic examination of the embryonic disc shows it to consist of three elements: the notochordal nucleus pulposus encapsulated by the annulus fibrosus and cartilaginous plates (Fig. 3.2).

The cartilaginous plates are "unossified epiphysis" of the vertebral bodies and are integral parts of the intervertebral discs. In the fetus and infant this envelope is highly vascular, being supplied by multiple capillary loops that never penetrate the nucleus, which remains totally avascular throughout life (Fig. 3.3).

As the person assumes adult erect life the pressure on the vertebra and disc becomes manifest. As the lordosis forms, the fluid nucleus pulposus migrates forward and changes shape, displacing the softer fibrocartilage that separated it from the anterior annular fibers. At 3 to 5 years of age the nucleus is large, soft, and viscous, and lies central within the disc.

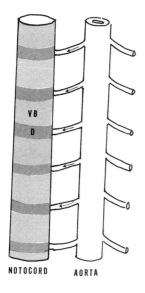

FIG. 3.1. Notochord-forming vertebrae and discs. The notochord is differentiated into dark and light bands. Each is at a branch of the primary aorta. The dark bands become intervertebral discs and the light bands the vertebral bodies. VB, vertebral body.

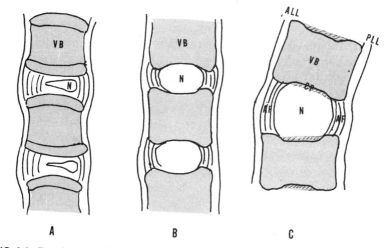

FIG. 3.2. Developmental stages of the intervertebral disc. The infant disc (**A**), the adolescent disc (**B**), and the adult disc (**C**). AF, annulus fibrosus; NP, nucleus pulposus; PLL, posterior longitudinal ligament; VB, vertebral body.

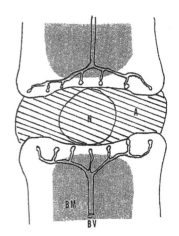

FIG. 3.3. Blood supply to the disc. The arteries (BV) end in small, bulblike endings near the endplate of the vertebra that are adjacent to the disc. In early life they penetrate the disc annulus (A) but never the nucleus (N). The blood vessels are in the bone marrow (BM) of the vertebrae.

During development of the erect posture the weight-bearing changes the shape of the components. The endplates change from convex or flat to a central concavity, being at the centrum of the disc nucleus.

By adult life the outer annular fibers are anchored to the bony rim and the inner lamellae are continuous with the cartilaginous plates. The outer lamellae are indistinguishable from the longitudinal ligaments. The anterior and lateral aspects of the annulus become thicker than the posterior portion and hence more resistant to changes of internal pressure.

The collagen fibers of the nucleus that have been considered as "random" have been shown to have orientation. The fibers near the cartilage plates are parallel to the plate and those deeper in the nucleus are convex inward, toward the center of the nucleus.

In the nucleus pulposus a progressive increase in collagen occurs, with decrease in cells as a result of decrease in vascularity, which produces proteoglycans. Spaces in the body endplates permit vascular spaces of the vertebral body marrow to come in contact with the cartilaginous plates. This is the basis for hydration of the "avascular" disc from inhibition (4).

There is a reduced water content in the young adult nucleus from the 88% of the newborn to the 76% of the adult (5). The adult disc still has a high level of hydration and can still absorb more water, especially in the nucleus. As dehydration occurs, for many reasons, numerous horizontal splits develop in the nucleus.

There is an existing pressure within the nucleus regardless of the external pressure on the disc. If the nucleus is sectioned, the disc narrows in an increased lordotic position and when it is reinjected with fluid resumes straightening. The clinical significance of this fact remains yet to be confirmed, but it appears to have an effect on the creep of vertebrae (6).

The annular fibers also vary in their alignment and density according to their position in the disc. In the anterior portion there are 20 fairly thick lamellae with the outer layers running vertical and loosely fused with the anterior longitudinal ligament.

The posterior fibers, especially the posterolateral fibers, are much thinner and are fused with the posterior longitudinal ligament. Occasionally, blood vessels have been found between the ligament and the outer annular fibers.

The stress on the annular fibers of the disc, which are collagen fibers attached to their adjacent endplates, causes them to undergo extensibility, which, when physiologic, retracts on cessation but when excessive or repetitive ends up with damage to the continuity of the fibers (7,8).

During development all cells are not removed from the disc in spite of its avascularity. There are varying cell densities as well as cell types within the disc. The annular fibers near the cartilage have the most numerous cells and the nucleus has the least. The nucleus contains notochordal and connective-tissue cells with the appearance of chondrocytes and fibroblasts dependent on the age of the person. Notochordal tissues and chondrocytes increase during fetal life and early childhood and decrease with aging.

The remnants of cells within the disc retain the ability to regenerate and repair the matrix. Determining the regenerative potential remains very difficult but has been made possible by immunohistochemical studies.

A recent article (9) has stated that mechanical stress on nucleus pulposus cells promotes proliferation of cells and their properties. This indicates that mechanical stresses on the disc have physiologic benefit in daily adaptation. Daily activities may be therapeutic in decreasing degenerative changes in normal discs.

COLLAGENOUS PLATES

At the periphery of each cartilaginous plate there is a ring apophysis that calcifies and persists in the adult vertebra, as does the central cartilaginous plate. The collagen fibers of the cartilaginous plate run parallel to the vertebral body. It is through this cartilaginous plate that diffusion nutrition to the disc occurs.

The stress on the annular fibers of the disc causes them to undergo varying degrees of elongation, depending on the movement of the functional unit (Fig. 3.4).

The nerve roots as they emerge from the spinal canal to the foramina are in direct contact with the posterolateral aspect of the disc. The

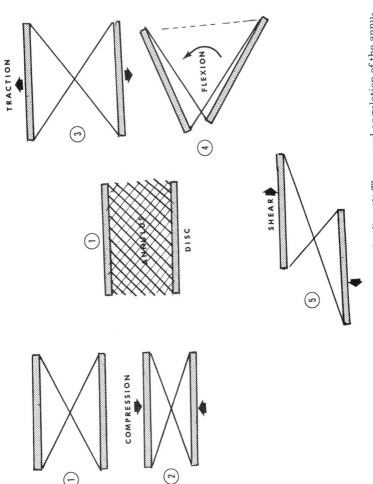

FIG. 3.4. Extensibility of the annular fibers of the disc. (1) The normal angulation of the annular fibers (2) under compression, (3) under traction, (4) during flexion and extension, and (5) under shear stress.

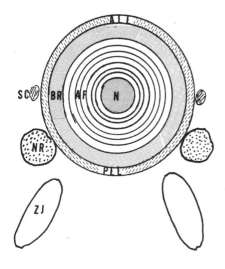

FIG. 3.5. Nerve relationship to intervertebral disc. The disc contains the nucleus (N), annular fibers (AF) contained within the bony ridge (BR). The anterior (ALL) and posterior (PLL) longitudinal ligaments surround the outer annular fibers. The nerve roots (NR) are located in the posterolateral aspect of the canal adjacent to the disc. SC, sympathetic nerve chain; ZJ, zygapophyseal joint.

sympathetic chain descends on the posterolateral surface of the disc. These anatomic relationships are vital to understanding pathologic changes that occur after injury (Fig. 3.5) (9,10).

The pathogenesis of intervertebral discs causing pain and impairment remains controversial. What is seen in a degenerated disc is progressive fraying and tearing of the annular fibers and dehydration of the nucleus.

Tears of the annulus have been classified into three types: (a) radiating tears seen most frequently in the posterolateral aspects of the discs, (b) concentric tears seen especially in the periphery but in all layers of the disc, and (c) discrete peripheral tears near the rim, termed *rim lesions.* The first detailed description of the morphology of "internal derangement of the intervertebral disc structure" was made by Schmorl and Junghann, who described clefts extending from the nucleus pulposus into the annular layers with a transverse or oblique course. They described lesions consistent with separation of the annulus fibrosus from the vertebral body rim along a plane parallel and adjacent to the endplate and seen specifically at the very periphery of the disc. Concentric fissuring of the annular lamellae were considered as normal aging from age 30 (11,12) (Fig. 3.6).

Rim lesions have been attributed to direct trauma rather than to degeneration, as they are common by age 20 (13,14). The most commonly accepted forces that damage the intervertebral disc are torsional (15,16).

The presence of a highly hydrated nucleus causes tensile strain on the surrounding annular fibers, which when damaged undergo

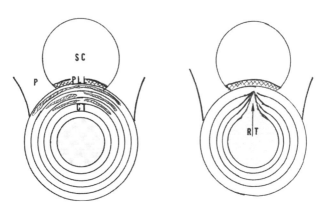

FIG. 3.6. Concentric and radial tears of the annulus. CT: Concentric tears of the annulus that essentially separate the annular sheets, causing weakness in their integrity. RT: Disruptions in the annular fibers allow extrusion of the nucleus radial tears. P, pedicle; SC, spinal column; PLL, posterior longitudinal ligament.

progressive deformation of the nucleus with bulging and dissection of its containing annular fibers. The hydrodynamics of the disc become defective.

Compression causes deformation but deformation is significantly greater from torque forces. This indicates that significant compressive forces are not borne by the outer annular fibers but instead are borne by the nucleus and the inner annular fibers (17).

The exact mechanism by which a disc prolapse occurs clinically remains undetermined, but numerous attempts at causing prolapse in vitro have revealed the following:

1. Compressive forces at high speed or slow speed result in fractures of the endplates but *not* in failure of the disc. This is true irrespective of the degree of disc degeneration (18–20).
2. Torsional loading of the disc beyond its physiologic limits results in tearing of the circumferential disc annulus but does not cause disc prolapse (15).
3. Excessive or abrupt flexion of the functional unit generally results in tearing of the posterior ligaments or avulsion fracture of the laminae.

At the ages of 40 to 50 years disc degeneration progresses. The nucleus remains mobile and therefore at a risk of prolapse, but the third stage is one of return of stabilization by virtue of ligament calcification and formation of osteophytes.

Clinically, most patients do not usually attribute their prolapse to a specific precipitating traumatic event. Therefore it behooves the clinician to get a careful detailed history that is related to the event alleged to have caused the clinical picture of low back pain and/or radiating leg pain. The diagnosis of disc prolapse therefore must be considered as the result of a combination of many factors: a weakened posterior disc annulus from multiple subclinical events that ultimately results in an acute prolapse from a flexion–rotational–compressive force.

Pathologic spines reveal that degenerative changes of the intervertebral disc are present in all subjects by middle age but are more marked at an earlier age when there is evidence of vertical or posterior disc prolapse. Disc degeneration ultimately leads to all the sequelae of degenerative spondylosis that become the diagnostic label of many pathologic states of low back pain and impairment (16–22).

The gelatinous matrix of the nucleus pulposus has been stated to contain a large number of proteoglycan complexes that have an affinity for water. Approximately 65% of its dry weight is accounted for by proteoglycan; 20%, by collagen; and the rest, by elastin and other minor components. The dry weight of the annulus is approximately 60% collagen and 20% proteoglycans. There are elastic fibers throughout the disc.

Since dehydration is claimed as a cause of disc degeneration the mechanism of this dehydration must be clarified. Proteoglycans decrease, along with a simultaneous increase in keratin sulfate. Neutral proteinases degrade cartilage matrix. Where these destructive enzymes are derived remains unclear, but they are currently found in vertebral bodies and thus probably flow into the disc matrix after trauma (23–26).

NUCLEAR MATERIAL CAUSING NOCICEPTION

When there is internal herniation within the disc, the nucleus protrudes outward and chemical changes occur within the matrix. Phospholipids A2 (PLA2) and glycoprotein elicit an autoimmune inflammatory reaction. The matrix of the nucleus normally contains PLA2 and PGI2, which is an end product of arachidonic acid. When the nucleus is damaged phospholipid A2 is released from arachidonic acid and becomes prostaglandin, thromboxane, leukotrienes, and lipozins, termed *eicosanoids,* which cause inflammation. The cells that are considered responsible for this cascade are the chondrocytes and fibroblasts (27–32).

That metabolites of arachidonic acid are involved in the production of local pain, and radicular pain is well confirmed (Fig. 3.7).

A combination of compression and torque causing disc annular tearing is compounded by lateral flexion, which never occurs without simultaneous rotation. With lateral flexion the opposing facets impact and become the axis about which rotation occurs. This changes

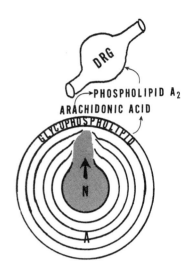

FIG. 3.7. Chemicals liberated from internal disc herniation. Internal herniation of the nucleus (N) is also accompanied by chemicals liberated from the damaged matrix. DRG, dorsal root ganglion.

the normal axis of rotation and thus causes a different force on the annular fibers (Fig. 3.8).

The role that the nucleus plays in production of low back pain and/or radiculitis has thus been ascertained to be chemical and mechanical. It has been postulated that when the disc material reaches the spinal canal or the foramen, it imbibes fluid to swell and compresses the neural tissues in the vicinity.

CLINICAL MANIFESTATIONS OF DISC DISEASE

The clinical picture of a herniated lumbar disc and its variations between protrusion and extrusions have been well defined, but the "diagnosis of the entity, the disc, as being the cause of the pain cannot be made on imaging tests alone in the absence of the clinical picture and/or findings at surgical intervention" (29,30).

Imaging techniques (myelogram, CT, MRI) should demonstrate actual nerve impingement at the precise level demonstrated by the clinical findings. The MRI may demonstrate "bulging" of the disc, but unless it is eccentric and actually displacing the nerve root it does not confirm the diagnosis of a herniated disc.

Discography with CT scanning may be more diagnostic of the disc as the culprit if the precise pain is reproduced. The dye injected must also extrude from the nucleus, confirming disc herniation from annular tears.

McKenzie (33,34) postulated migration of the nucleus, considered both diagnostic and therapeutic of disc herniation. So long as the

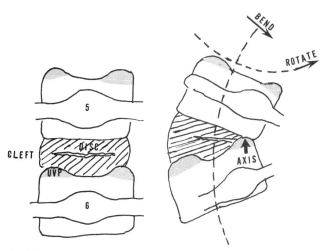

FIG. 3.8. Combined lateral flexion and rotation causing disc annular damage. This illustration is of the cervical spine, but a similar force occurs in the lumbar spine where there are no uncovertebral joints. The left figure shows the erect spine with a posterior annular tear. The right figure shows lateral flexion and rotation on the newly created axis of rotation. UVP, uncovertebral joints of the cervical spine.

annulus fibrosus remains intact and unaffected by static loading presented in everyday activities, the patient will experience no more than the postural low back pain frequently experienced and of short duration. The undamaged annulus fibrosus will retain the nucleus within its confines. With any defect in the annulus there is displacement and possibly degenerative chemical as well as mechanical changes causing pain.

As displacement progresses from repeated flexion injuries or an acute insult, pain increases and, according to McKenzie, moves distally. Movements applied to the damaged functional unit increase displacement. By increasing postural extension of the low back the disc nucleus is mechanically displaced posteriorly, away from the posterior longitudinal ligament and the nerve roots, and the pain subsides. The distal pain in the leg diminishes to merely low back pain, then, theoretically, disappears.

The importance of the disc has been accepted in its role of the mechanics of the lumbar spine and accepted as a site of pain, but confirmation that the disc is the cause must be achieved with an accurate clinical picture, history and physical examination, and confirmatory radiologic studies.

Those likely to develop discogenic disease are difficult to determine because the environmental and anthropometric risk factors are modest, although a genetic factor has been suggested.

In his provocative article (35), Adams suggests that the mechanical mechanism of disc disruption is as follows: with a damaged endplate a load deforms the plate, allowing the nucleus to penetrate it. This decreases the intradiscal pressure and allows narrowing of the disc space and hence a loss in stability as the pressure is borne by the annulus rather than the nucleus. Thus stress on the annulus forces the inner annular fibers to bulge inwardly and the outer annular fibers to bulge outwardly.

The resultant instability from progressive damage to the disc, the posterior facet joints, and the neurologic damage to the nerve tissues within the foramen can only be prevented or minimized by improving the "tubular" support of the vertebral column, which is advocated in the treatment chapter.

SUMMARY

The role of the disc in the mechanics of the spine has been accepted, and it has been accepted as a nociceptive site as well. The history and physical examination do not usually describe the actual pathomechanism, nor do radiologic and magnetic resonance studies (MRI) clearly associate the history with the clinical finding, as abnormal radiologic findings are found with no clinical findings. The disc is merely assumed to be the culprit in many of the impairing painful conditions that present to the clinician (36).

REFERENCES

1. Taylor JR, Twomey L. The role of the notochord and blood vessels in vertebral column development and in the aetiology of Schmorl's nodes. In: Grieve GP, ed. *Modern manual therapy of the vertebral column.* Edinburgh: Churchill Livingstone, 1986:2–26.
2. Taylor JR. The development and adult structure of lumbar intervertebral discs. *J Man Med* 1990;5:43–47.
3. Peacock A. Observations on the prenatal development of the intervertebral disc in man. *J Anat* 1951;85:260–274.
4. Maroudas A, Stockwell RA, Nachemson A, et al. Factors involved in the nutrition of the human intervertebral disc. *J Anat* 1975;120:113–130.
5. Puschel J. Der Wassergehalt normaler und degenerierter Zwiaschenwirbelsheiben. *Beitr Pathol Anat* 1930;84:123–126.
6. Twomey L, Taylor J., Flexion creep deformation and hysteresis in the lumbar column. *Spine* 1982;7:116–122.
7. Paassilta P, et al. Identification of a novel common genetic risk factor for lumbar disk disease. *JAMA* 2001;285:1843–1849.
8. Marini JC. Genetic risk factors for lumbar disk disease. *JAMA* 2001;285 1886–1888.

9. Bogduk N, Tynan W, Wilson AS. The nerve supply to the human lumbar intervertebral discs. *J Anat* 1981:132:39–56.

10. Taylor J, Twomey L. Innervation of lumbar intervertebral discs. *NZ J Physiother* 1980;8:36–37.

11. Matsumoto T, Kawakami M, Kuribayashi K, et al. Cyclic mechanical stretch stress increases the growth rate and collagen synthesis of nucleus pulposus cells in vitro. *Spine* 1999;24:4:315–319.

12. Schmorl G, Junghann H. *The human spine in health and disease.* Second American Edition. Besemann EF, trans. New York: Grune & Stratton, 1971.

13. Coventry MB, Ghormley RK, Kernohan JW. The intervertebral disc: its microscopic anatomy and pathology. Part III: Pathological changes in the intervertebral disc. *J Bone Joint Surg* 1945;27:460.

14. Friberg S. Anatomical studies on lumbar disc degeneration. *Acta Orthop Scand* 1948;17:224–230.

15. Vernon-Roberts B, Fraser RD. Annular tears and intervertebral disc degeneration. *Spine* 1990;15:762–767.

16. Vernon Roberts B, Pirie CJ. Degenerative changes in the intervertebral discs of the lumbar spine and their sequelae. *Rheumatol Rehab* 1977; 16:13–21.

17. Farfan HF. *Mechanical disorders of the low back.* Philadelphia: Lea & Febiger, 1973:63–92.

18. Kirkaldy-Willis WH. The pathology and pathogenesis of low back pain. In: Kirkaldy-Willis WH, ed. *Managing low back pain.* New York: Churchill-Livingstone, 1983:23–43.

19. White AA, Panjabi MM. *Clinical biomechanics of the spine,* 2nd ed. Philadelphia: JB Lippincott, 1990:16.

20. Hardy WG, Lissner HR, Webster JE, et al. Repeated loading tests of the lumbosacral spine. *Surg Forum* 1958;9:690.

21. Perry O. Fracture of the vertebral end-plate in the lumbar spine. *Acta Orthop Scand* 1957(Suppl);25.

22. Virgin W. Experimental investigations into physical properties of intervertebral disc. *J Bone Joint Surg* 1951;33B:607.

23. Roaf R. A study of the mechanics of spinal injuries. *J Bone Joint Surg* 1960;42B:810.

24. Adams MA, Hutton WC. Prolapsed intervertebral disc: hyperflexion injury. *Spine* 1982;7:184.

25. Shirazi-Adl A, Parianpor M. Effect of changes in lordosis on mechanics of the lumbar spine-lumbar curvature in lifting. *J Spinal Disord* 1999; 12:436–447.

26. Gracovetsky S. *The spinal engine.* New York: Springer-Verlag, 1988.

27. Fujita K, Nakagawa T, Hirabayashi K, et al. Neutral proteinases in human intervertebral discs role in degeneration and probable origin. *Spine* 1993;18:1766–1773.

28. Paajanen H, Haapasalo H, Kotilainen E, et al. Proliferation potential of human lumbar disc after herniation. *J Spinal Disord* 1999;12:57–60.

29. Brown MD. Pathophysiology of disc disease. *Orthop Clin North Am* 1971;2:359–370.

30. Robertson JT, Huffmon GV, Thomas LB, et al. Prostaglandin production after experimental discectomy. *Spine* 1996;21:1731–1736.

31. Shimizu T, Wolfe LS. Arachidonic acid cascade and signal transduction. *J Neurochem* 1990;55:1–15.

32. Gertzbein SD, Tile M, Gross A, et al. Autoimmunity in degenerative disc disease of the lumbar spine. *Orthop Clin North Am* 1975:6:67–73.
33. McKenzie R. A physical therapy perspective on acute spinal disorders. In: Mayer TG, Mooney V, Gatchel RJ, eds. *Contemporary conservative care for painful spinal disorders.* Philadelphia: Lea & Febiger, 1991: 211–220.
34. McKenzie R. *The cervical and thoracic spine: mechanical diagnosis and therapy.* Waikanae, NZ: Spinal Publications, 1989.
35. Adams MA, Freeman BJC, Morrison HP, et al. Mechanical initiation of intervertebral disc degeneration. *Spine* 2000;25:1625–1636.
36. Laros GS. Differential diagnosis of low back pain. In: Mayer TG, Mooney V, Gatchel RJ, eds. *Contemporary care for painful spinal disorders.* Philadelphia: Lea & Febiger, 1991:122–130.

4. THE ROLE OF THE FACETS IN LOW BACK PAIN

The zygapophyseal joints (also known as *facets*) are synovial joints located in the laminar aspect of the functional unit. Sagittally placed, they allow flexion and extension of the spine but markedly limit lateral flexion and rotation of the functional units (Fig. 4.1).

Besides guiding the movement of the vertebral functional unit, they have numerous nerve end organs that function as proprioceptors and as nociceptors in the presence of inflammation (1). Proprioceptor end organs have been verified within the deep back muscles, tendons, interspinous ligament, and the facets, and provide information as to movement. Nociception implies that inflammation and injury transmit pain to the central nervous system. These nerve end organs are also present in the posterior ligamentous structures as well as in the facets (Fig. 4.2).

Because of this innervation they are also considered a major site of low back pain. In 1911 Goldthwait stated, "the peculiarities of the facets were responsible for low back pain and instability" (2). The term *facet joint syndrome* was added to the taxonomy of low back pain when it was discovered that pain could be elicited by a noxious injection into the joint and was relieved by subsequent injection of an analgesic agent (3). Numerous articles have been subsequently written confirming this finding (4).

At the outermost range of flexion of the functional unit the facet joint capsule comes under tension, providing resistance to further flexion (5,6).

By the angulation of the facets they limit rotation, lateral flexion, and translatory shear motion (Fig. 4.3). This limitation further ensures stability of the functional unit, along with the ligaments and disc annular fibers.

Being synovial joints, their lubrication is made possible because their opposing surfaces are lined with cartilage. The cartilaginous lining averages 1 mm thick. The cartilage, being avascular, gets its nutrition and lubrication material from imbibition of subchondral blood vessels.

Lubrication of the joint also serves to minimize compressive forces. Mechanisms such as lubrication are possible because of the mechanical structure of the cartilage. The normal secretion of cartilage is hyaluronidase, which is the lubricant of a synovial joint. This secretion is expressed into the joint by compressive forces of gravity and muscular contraction. It minimizes friction by coating the joint surfaces with its adhesive properties.

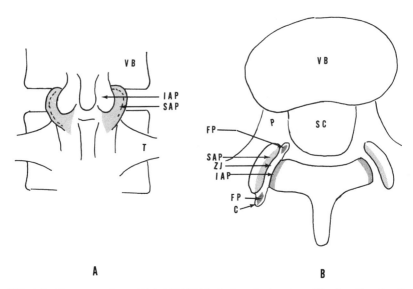

FIG. 4.1. The zygapophyseal joint (FACET). **A:** A posterior view of the functional units depicting the zygapophyseal (facet) joints. **B:** A superior view showing the facets. C, capsule; FP, fat pads; IAP, inferior articular process; P, pedicle; SAP superior articular process; SC, spinal canal; T, transverse processes; VB, vertebral bodies; Z-J, zygapophyseal joint.

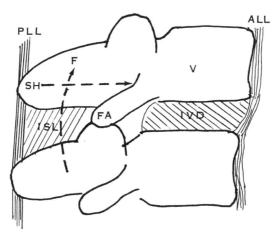

FIG. 4.2. Interspinous ligaments. A side view of a functional unit reveals the posterior spinous ligament (PLL), interspinous ligaments (ISL), anterior longitudinal ligament (ALL) that determine the movements of the unit vertebrae (V): flexion (F) and shear (SH). FA, facets; IVD, intervertebral disc.

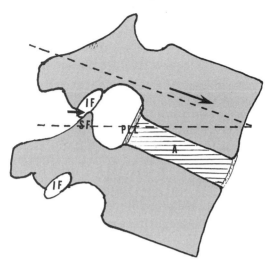

FIG. 4.3. Facet prevention of shear motion. From the lumbosacral angle that would permit shear motion, the angulation of the facets prevents significant translatory motion (*small arrows*).

Degeneration of cartilage occurs from repeated and/or excessive forces imposed upon the cartilage. Narrowing of the intervertebral disc anteriorly in the functional unit places abnormal forces upon the facets located posteriorly that can damage the cartilage. These forces involve compression with and without excessive shear. Usually there is a combination of these forces (7).

Degradation of the cartilage means a change in the matrix as well as damage to the collagen fibers. This occurs because of chemical release of proteolytic enzymes from the damaged chondrocytes, synovial cells, and neutrophils (8–10). These proteinases are also termed *collagenases,* as they also destroy collagen. They are also termed *stromelysin,* because they destroy matrix, and termed *elastase,* as they destroy elastin.

Degeneration of cartilage is believed to result from

1. Longitudinal forces from muscular contraction and other external forces.
2. Excessive compressive forces upon the cartilage, also from muscular contraction and external forces.
3. Acute impact upon the subchondral bone, causing microfractures (11).
4. Excessive shear forces from inadvertent motion of the spine (12,13).

Stress as a physical stimulus is a significant factor in the formation and maintenance of collagen (14). Abnormal stresses cause degeneration and aging.

Damage to a cartilage that does not reach the subchondral tissues does not get worse, nor does it improve. Initial degeneration occurs as a "flaking" of the superficial surface of the cartilage, forming small cysts in the tangential layers. Hyaluronidase enters these craters and damages the chondroitin of the cartilage matrix.

With progressive degenerative changes the elasticity of the cartilage decreases. Less lubricant is formed, allowing more friction upon movement. Fibroblasts from the subchondral bone enter the cartilage fissures, increasing the degree of bone, with ultimate movement occurring as bone against bone rather than as cartilage against cartilage.

During flexion-extension of a functional unit the facets glide up and down on each other with some compression and some shear. The capsule elongates physiologically but may tear when the force is excessive as the facets disengage. In forward flexion the facets undergo a slight degree of translation (shear) of up to 3 mm. This amount of shear is considered physiologic as limited by the annular fibers, the capsule of the facets, the posterior longitudinal ligament, and the thoracolumbar fascia of the muscles.

Forward flexion during most activities of daily living is accompanied by simultaneous rotation and lateral flexion, as there is rarely pure sagittal flexion and extension (15). Each functional unit therefore undergoes simultaneous flexion, lateral flexion, and rotation during spinal flexion. The facets glide upon each other with some compression and some shear. During these movements the capsule elongates physiologically.

Fat pads within the folds of the capsule add to the congruity of the joint and thus to their lubrication (16,17). These pads are lined with synovium and in older people become fibrotic and lose their elasticity and thus their lubricating potential (18–20).

FACET JOINT INNERVATION

The facet joints are innervated by the posterior primary division of the nerve roots and contain afferent and efferent nerves as well as sympathetic nerve fibers. Their function is sensorimotor, proprioceptive, and vasomotor control (Fig. 4.4).

The proprioceptive function of the facets has been assumed to be significant in the spontaneous reduction of myoelectric activity in the lumbar erector spinae muscles (ESM) during flexion activities (5,6) (Fig. 4.5).

The accumulation of nociceptors at the end organs of the sensory fibers also sensitizes the dorsal root ganglion fibers, causing them to initiate further impulses to the dorsal horn neurons. Further or sustained inflammation at the periphery is no longer necessary, as the dorsal root neurons and the dorsal horn neurons now become the primary sites of nociception (Fig. 4.6).

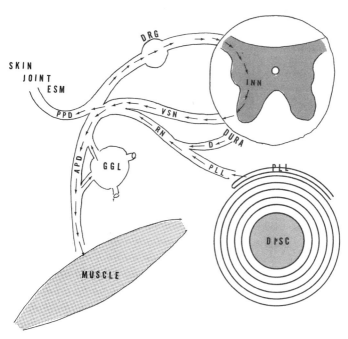

FIG. 4.4. Innervation of facets (joint). The innervation of all the nociceptive sites including the joint from the posterior primary division (PPD) are shown. APD, anterior primary division; D, dural; DRG, dorsal root ganglion; ESM, extensor spinal muscles; GGL, sympathetic ganglion; INN, internuncial nerves; PLL, posterior longitudinal ligament; RN, recurrent nerve Luschka; VSN, ventral sensory nerve.

DEGENERATIVE FACET DISEASE

When there is discogenic disease that narrows the anterior compartment of the functional unit there is simultaneous narrowing of the posterior elements, especially the facets that undergo degenerative changes with bony hypertrophy. This causes stenosis of the foramen with possible entrapment of the nerve root at that level (Fig. 4.7).

Radiologic studies such as oblique X-rays, CT scanning, and MRI studies will reveal the presence and degree of foramenal narrowing, and MRI studies may reveal nerve root entrapment. Electromyographic evaluations may confirm the specific nerve root entrapped and the degree of neural damage but do not per se ascertain that the stenosis is the pathoanatomic basis of nerve root entrapment.

CLINICAL MANIFESTATIONS OF FACET DISEASE

Ascertaining the facets as being the source of pain and impairment remains controversial and difficult to confirm. The standard tests for confirming pain arising from the facets is active and passive hyper-

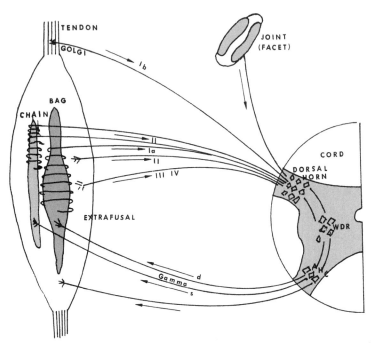

FIG. 4.5. Relationship of facet inflammation to muscle spasm. Inflammation of the facet joint sends impulses to the dorsal horn of the cord that progress to the wide dynamic range nuclei (WDR) that initiate impulses to the anterior horn cells (AHC), which cause contraction of the extrafusal muscle fibers. They also disrupt the intrafusal: bag and chain of the spindle system, resulting in a sustained muscular contraction termed *spasm*.

extension of the patient's low back with simultaneous lateral flexion to both sides. This maneuver approximates the facets narrowing the foramina and entrapping the nerve roots. Reproduction of the patient's symptom alludes to the facets as the culprit (21,22).

Injection of an analgesic agent into the facets joint is considered diagnostic and often therapeutic (23–27).

Ascertaining that the facets are the site and source of low back pain, impairment, or a contribution to sciatic radiculopathy remains very difficult, if even possible. Mere relief from an analgesic injection does not confirm that the facet is the cause, as it must be remembered that a facet does not receive just one specific nerve root branch but is innervated by two nerve root levels (27,28).

The foramina get narrowed from degenerative changes: anteriorly from the vertebral spurs and posteriorly from the facet arthritic changes (Fig. 4.8).

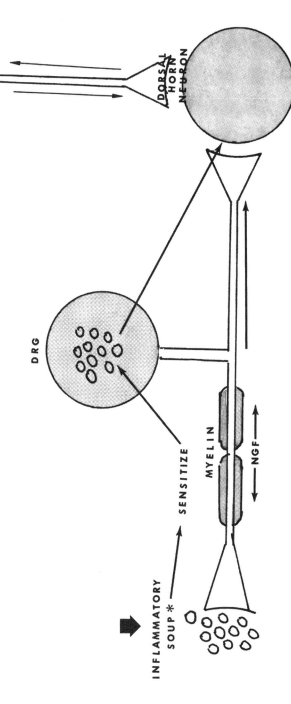

FIG. 4.6. Inflammatory "soup" concept. Accumulation of nociceptor chemicals at the end organs of the sensory nerves, termed *soup*, sensitizes the neurons of the dorsal root ganglion (DRG) neurons, then the neurons of the dorsal horn, causing persistence of inflammation no longer needing peripheral nociception, thus "chronic pain." *, glutamate, NMDA, substance P, etc.

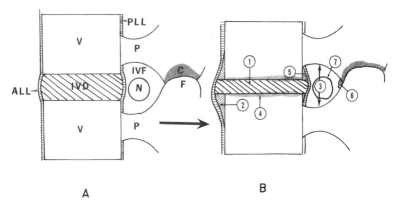

FIG. 4.7. Evolution of facet degenerative arthritis. (A) Shows the normal relationships of all elements within the functional unit; (B) Degenerative changes: (1) narrowing of the disc, (2) calcification of the hemorrhagic infiltration of the space where the longitudinal ligament is separated from the vertebra, (3) narrowing of the foramen, (4) thickening of the plate, (5) posterior osteophyte, (6) thickening of the facet cartilage and (7) subsequent narrowing of the foramen from (5) and (6). ALL, anterior longitudinal ligament; C, cartilage; F, facet; IVD, intervertebral disc; N, nerve; P, pedicle; PLL, posterior longitudinal ligament; V, vertebra.

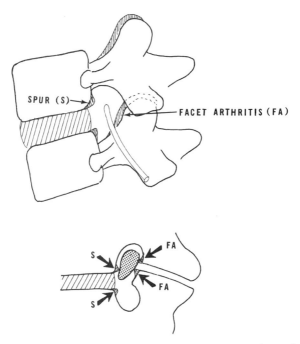

FIG. 4.8. Degenerative changes affecting the foramen. Spurs (S) on the posterior surfaces of the vertebra and the arthritic changes of the facets (FA) narrow the foramen and compress the nerve root.

Continued degeneration of the facets results in more instability of the functional unit with more shear. This may cause listhesis (forward shear movement).

REFERENCES

1. Minaki Y, Yamashita T, Ishii S. An electrophysiological study on the mechanoreceptors in the lumbar spine and adjacent tissues. *Neuro-Orthopedics* 1996;20:23–35.
2. Goldthwait JE. The lumbosacral articulations: an explanation of many cases of lumbago, sciatica, and paraplegia. *Boston Med Surg J* 1911; 164:365.
3. Mooney V, Robertson J. The facet syndrome. *Clin Orthop* 1976;115:149.
4. Cailliet R. *Low back pain syndrome,* 5th ed. Philadelphia: FA Davis, 1996.
5. Taylor JB, Twomey LT. Structure and function of lumbar zygapophyseal (facet) joints: a review. *J Orthoped Med* 1992;14:71.
6. Adams MA, Hutton W. The mechanical function of the lumbar joints. *Spine* 1983;8:327.
7. Giles L, Taylor JR. Human zygapophyseal joint capsule and synovial fold innervation. *Br J Rheumatol* 1987;26:93.
8. Ghosh P, Andrews JL, Osborne R, et al. Variations with aging and degeneration of serine and cysteine proteinase inhibitors of human cartilage. *Agents Actions* 1986;18:69–81.
9. Nakagawa T, Ghosh P, Nagai Y. Serine proteinase and serine proteinase inhibitors of normal and degenerate knee joint menisci. *Bio Med Res* 1983;4:25.
10. Melrose J, Ghosh P. The noncollagenous proteins of the intervertebral disc. In: Ghosh P, ed. *The biology of the intervertebral disc,* vol 1. Boca Raton, Fl: CRC Press, 1988:189–237.
11. Sellier N, Chevrot A, Vallee C, et al. Arthrographie vertebrale normale. *J Radiol* 1986;67:487–495.
12. Twomey LT, Taylor JR. Zygapophyseal joints of the lumbar spine. *Proceedings of 5th Biennial Congress of the Manipulative Therapist Association of Australia,* 1988.
13. Taylor JR, Twomey LT. Age changes in lumbar zygapophyseal joints: observations on structure and function. *Spine* 1986;11:739–745.
14. Tillman LJ, Cummings GS. Biological mechanisms of connective tissue mutability. In: Currier DP, Nelson RM, eds. *Dynamics of human biological tissues.* Philadelphia: FA Davis, 1992:1–44.
15. Lorenzm, Parwardhan A, Vanderby R. Load-bearing characteristics of lumbar facets in normal and surgically altered spinal segments. *Spine* 1983;8:122.
16. Fritz JM, Delitto A, Welch WC, et al. Lumbar spinal stenosis: a review of current concepts in evaluation, management, and outcome measurements. *Arch Phys Med Rehabil* 1998;79:700–708.
17. Taylor JR, McCormick CC. Lumbar facet joint fat pads: their normal anatomy and their appearance when enlarged. *Neuroradiology* 1991; 33:38.
18. Mankon HJ. The reaction of articular cartilage to injury and osteoarthritis: medical progress. *N Engl J Med* 1974;291:1335.
19. Polle AR. Enzymic degradation: cartilage destruction. In: Brandt KD, ed. *Cartilage changes in osteoarthritis.* Indianapolis: Indiana University Medical School of Medicine, 1990.

20. Giles L, Taylor JRT. Human zygapophyseal joint capsule and synovial fold innervation. *Br J Rheumatol* 1987;26:93–98.
21. Laros GS. Differential diagnosis of low back pain. In: Mayer TG, Mooney V, Gatchel RJ, eds. *Contemporary conservative care for painful spinal disorders,* Philadelphia: Lea & Febiger, 1991.
22. Maigne R., Le Corre F, Judet H. Lumbalgies basses d'origine dorso-lombaire: traitement chirurgical par excision des capsules articulaires postérieurs. Raport préliminaire. *Nouvelle Presse Med* 1978;7:565.
23. Lynch MC, Taylor JF. Facet joint injection for low back pain: a clinical study. *J Bone Joint Surg (Br)* 1986;68:138.
24. Marks RC, Houston T, Thulbourne F. Facet joint injection and facet nerve block: a randomized comparison in 86 patients with chronic low back pain. *Pain* 1992;49:325.
25. Carrera GF. Lumbar facet joint injection in low back pain and sciatica: description of technique. *Radiology* 1980;137:661.
26. Bogduk N, Long DM. The anatomy of the so-called "articular nerves" and their relationship to facet denervation in the treatment of low back pain. *J Neurosurg* 1979;51:172.
27. Bogduk N, Long DM. Percutaneous medial branch neurotomy: a modification of facet denervation. *Spine* 1980;5:193–200.

5. MUSCULAR CONTROL OF THE LOW BACK

The functional role of the spinal muscles has been discussed in previous chapters. As stated by Ladin (1), "Muscles balance the external movements in response to external loads." Other vertebral tissues, such as ligaments, tendons, and joint capsules, assist in equilibrium and balancing the muscular forces. "The smallest possible muscle forces that satisfy the moment equilibrium equations and minimize spinal compression forces are the physiological needs of activity" (1).

A disorder of muscle function that leads to impairment, disability, and pain is a neurophysiologic manifestation. The normal neural mechanisms are inherent, then modified by training and repetitive use, become "automatic" unless altered by "perturbers." These perturbers of normal neuromusculoskeletal function are numerous and include fatigue, boredom, anger, impatience, anxiety, distraction, and fear of recurrence of injury (Fig. 5.1).

The coupling motions of the spine, such as combined flexion, lateral flexion, and rotation, all, to a varying degree, compound the intricate muscle mechanisms. The simultaneous relaxation of antagonists as agonists contract at a specific speed and force also compound the intricacies of muscular activities (Fig. 5.2).

By faulty neuromuscular activity the other tissues of the functional unit—the intervertebral disc, the ligaments, and the facets—may be exposed to mechanical trauma with resultant impairment, disability, and pain. As has been stated, the vertebral column devoid of its muscles is unstable (2). With improper muscular activity the stability is not adequately restored and maintained. Any additional load may therefore displace the spine.

The muscles that directly control the movements of the vertebral column are divided into categories according to their relationship to the spine: postvertebral and prevertebral. The postvertebral are further divided into three groups: deep, intermediate, and superficial.

The deep muscles consist of short muscles that connect adjacent spinous processes: posterior and transverse. The intermediate also attach from the transverse processes to the posterior spinous processes. The superficial muscles are collectively called the *erector spinae* and are long, without segmental attachments.

The prevertebral muscles are the four abdominal muscles, of which three encircle the abdominal region: external oblique, internal oblique, and transversus. The fourth is the rectus abdominis, which lies vertically anteriorly in the midline. The spinal muscles produce body movements by generating bending forces and torques, and

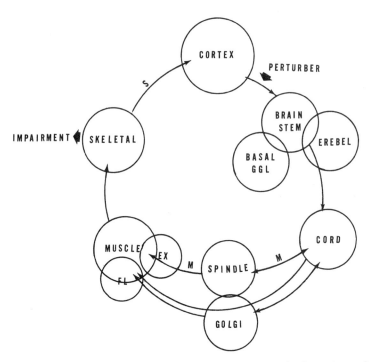

FIG. 5.1. Motor cortex patterns. The motor patterns originate in the cortex and the brain stem and are transmitted to the spinal cord for resultant muscular activities. The muscles are coordinated by the spindle system and the Golgi apparatus innervated by Ia and Ib fibers. External forces are apparent and internal forces are perturbers. M, motor nerves; S, sensory nerve.

resist external forces. They produce stability by reinforcing the ligamentous spine.

Muscles generate force isometrically as well as isotonically, depending on the activity required. All muscular contractions are guided by the intrinsic systems—the spindle and Golgi apparatus—and have a sensory component.

Impaired function with or without resultant pain is determined clinically by evaluating active and passive movements, described in Chapter 2.

SPASM

Muscle "spasm," which permeates the literature and clinical reports, allegedly results as a sequela of inflammation of tissue within the vertebral column. *Spasm* is rarely discussed, defined, documented, or given a neurophysiologic basis. In a review of numerous texts the term is mentioned but never defined. It must be assumed that in-

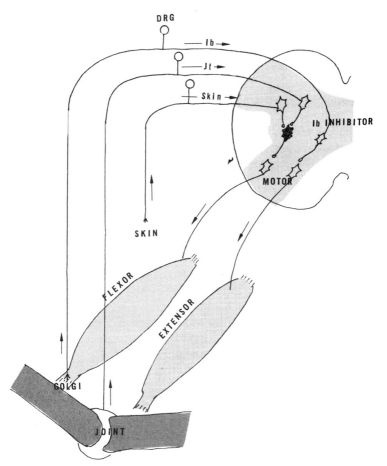

FIG. 5.2. Agonist–antagonistic muscular contraction. As an agonist muscle contracts (flexor) the antagonist relaxes (extensor). Impulses from the Golgi via Ib fibers synapse with inhibitor nuclei (Ib) that influence the antagonist. Sensory fibers from the joint capsule via (Jt) have an influential effect.

flammation within the functional unit causes an isometric contraction of the adjacent muscles to prevent further motion that may aggravate the pain. Interestingly, there has never been a documented electromyographic verification of this "protective spasm."

DeVries, in his *Physiology of Exercise,* is the only author, in my literature research, that discusses spasm; he states, "There are two major theoretical positions with respect to the causation of delayed muscle soreness: the muscle spasm theory and the structural damage theory" (3). His "spasm theory" is suggested by observation of typical muscle fatigue curves in exercised muscles. The addition of a decrement in amplitude of contraction with increasing fatigue causes a decrease in the ability of a muscle to relax completely. This allegedly causes a degree of ischemia, which causes pain, probably from a transfer of substance P across the muscle membrane, where it gains access to pain nerve endings. This pain brings about a reflex tonic muscle contraction that prolongs the muscle ischemia, resulting in a vicious cycle. This reflex tonic contraction occurs via the Golgi apparatus. This is verified by stretching the afflicted muscle. De Vries demonstrated electromyographic changes that were elicited from passive stretching of the contracted muscle. De Vries did his electromyographic studies with his devised instrument, which recorded integrated EMG potentials.

Marinacci (4) defined *benign muscle spasm* as a "fasciculation" having a wave form of three or four spikes with amplitude of 100 to 1,200 μV for 2 to 10 msec. It was considered benign, as it was not a sign of lower motor nerve degeneration. These physiologic definitions indicate that muscle "spasm" is a neurologic isometric contraction of muscles initiated by a painful incidence, which in turn becomes a painful condition due to ischemia. Passive stretching does afford relief. While maintained, this isometric muscle contraction diminishes passive and active range of motion of the joint involved—in this case the vertebral functional unit (Figs. 5.3 and 5.4).

A recent basis for muscle spasm has been expounded by Gunn, whose work has been set forth in his book (5). His concept is based on the concepts of Cannon and Rosenblueth's law of denervation (6). Cannon's law states, "When a unit is destroyed, in a series of efferent neurons, an increased irritability to chemical agents develops in the isolated structure or structures, the effect being maximal in the part denervated."

Gunn (5) termed "spasm" as increased muscle tension with (or without) muscle shortening "from a nonvoluntary motor nerve activity as continued motor unit activity." He further postulates that "there can be shortening of muscle fibers in the absence of action potential" but from denervation supersensitivity (6) of the muscle fibers, which are supersensitive to acetylcholine of the entire muscle fibers and not merely at their motor unit. He also states that "it is best to avoid using the term *spasm* when describing muscle shortening."

In his thesis he postulates that numerous musculoskeletal pain syndromes, of which low back disorders are one, are caused by this muscle shortening with increase in disc compression, approximation of the facets, and muscle ischemia. The concepts of Gunn deserve the statement by Patrick D. Wall in his foreword (5) that Gunn's concept envisions "profound understanding of anatomy and physiology of movement." Further clinical studies will evolve.

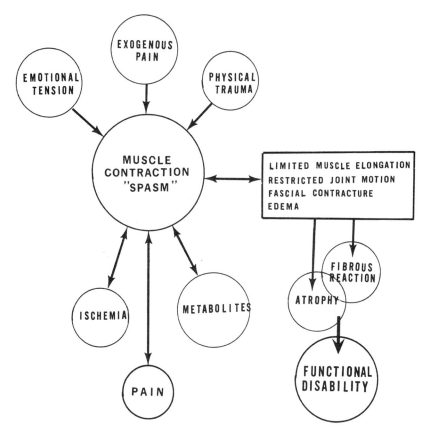

FIG. 5.3. Muscle spasm and functional disability. Trauma, exogenous pain, and emotional tension cause ischemia of the involved muscles from vasoconstriction- and edema-eliciting muscle spasm.

MYOGENIC PAIN

In a differential diagnosis of low back pain that included the disc, ligaments, and facet capsule, Laros (7) included *myogenic pain.* This term was included with others such as *myositis, fibromyositis,* and *myofascial syndrome,* but myogenic pain can occur as an expected sequela of any of the other injuries to the tissues of the functional unit and become a painful entity in itself.

Noxious impulses have been found to be mediated through the motor fibers going to the muscle; therefore the term *muscular pain* has a structural basis (8) (Fig. 5.5).

Clinically, the presence of muscle pathology reveals limited range of motion; local tenderness, usually in the paraspinous muscles and the glutei; reproduction of the pain by passive and active stretching;

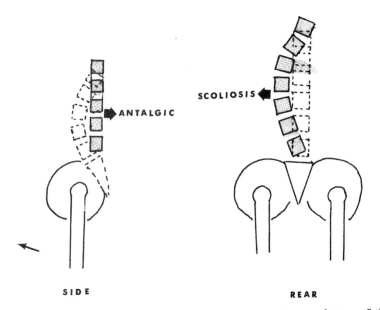

FIG. 5.4. Antalgia spine and functional scoliosis. In "protective muscle spasm" the spine loses its physiologic lordosis and straightens (side view). Unilateral muscle spasm may cause a "functional scoliosis" (rear view).

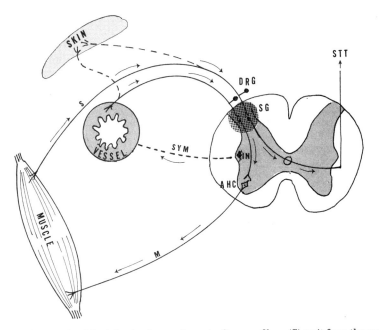

FIG. 5.5. Neurophysiologic basis of muscular pain. Sensory fibers (S) emit from the muscle that enters the dorsal root ganglion (DRG) and enter the substantia gelatinosum (SG). Then they ascend through the spinal thalamic tracts (STT) to the thalamus. Synaptic connection (IN) to the anterior horn cell (AHC) could contract the muscle (M). Blood vessels contract through sympathetic fibers (SYM) that assist in causing ischemia

and reproduction of pain by active contraction against resistance. The history may indicate possible muscle tearing by the violence of the act that caused the low back pain, but most injuries are not that excessive.

Muscle pain in the low back may also be palpated in the muscles of the myotome when a peripheral nerve has been damaged and made supersensitive (6,9). Palpation of tender muscle bands is diagnostic.

FATIGUE

Fatigue is the decreased capacity to produce tension or shortening resulting from prior activity. Human performance is adversely affected by fatigue. Fatigue has been aptly called a "transient loss of performance capacity resulting from preceding performance regardless of whether the current performance is affected" (10).

Fatigue may be central fatigue within the central nervous system or peripheral fatigue of the neuromusculoskeletal unit. Central fatigue may be neurologic organic disease or motivational and psychologic, whereas peripheral fatigue probably has a chemical basis. Fatigue may occur on the basis of defective motor–neuronal firing or be a depletion of muscle glycogen (10–13).

Fatigue is a contributing factor in the production of acute low back pain and can be considered a perturber in that it impairs the sequence of neuromusculoskeletal function. Thus the normal sequence of activities may be impaired and the improper sequence may strain the tissues within the functional unit.

MYALGIA

Strenuous physical activity is normally accompanied by a subjective sensation of fatigue that disappears rapidly after cessation of the activity. For those unaccustomed to exercise, however, localized muscle soreness is commonly experienced for some hours after exercise (14,15).

Eccentric muscle contraction is where the active muscle lengthens while doing its work. Histologic evidence exists of extensive disruption of muscle structure with lesions localized in the region of the Z-discs. Muscle strength can be reduced by about 50% after such exercise (16).

It must be remembered that the erector spinae muscles contract eccentrically in flexion activities as decelerating muscles. When done excessively and repeatedly, fatigue results. With a weakened muscle the other tissues of the functional unit, the discs especially, are exposed to excessive and inappropriate stress. Muscular pain also results in muscular irritation. In addition, the enclosing fascia and irritated and this becomes the site of noxious stimulation (17).

Trunk muscle endurance appears to be a better indicator of future low back pain than does strength. Fatigue indicates a significant decrease in motor performance in which the reduction in force-generating capability and the decline in speed of contraction produce greater loading on the passive tissues of the spine in the event of an unexpected perturbation in load or position. A change in muscle recruitment also takes place, with significant increase in contraction of internal oblique and latissimus dorsi muscles (18–20).

Pain in the muscle has undergone numerous studies since the prominence of fibromyalgia diagnosis. Fibromyalgia is "a syndrome characterized by chronic pain widely distributed through all skeletal muscles and soft tissues" (5). There are three syndromes:

1. *Primary fibromyalgia syndrome* (PFS): fibrositis or diffuse myofascial pain syndrome: also known as *primary diffuse fibrositis syndrome.*
2. *Myofascial pain syndrome* (MPS): considered to be a specific myofascial pain.
3. *Temporomandibular pain and dysfunction* (TMPDS).

Of the three if there is pain localized in the paraspinous muscle area it would fall in the MPS syndrome, but there would also need to be muscular pain elsewhere and with nodularity and the other symptoms of PFS.

CONCLUSION

The enigma of low back disorders can be clarified to some extent if the muscular aspect in the neuromusculoskeletal system is fully understood. What is assumed is informative as to what impairs musculoskeletal function and causes symptomatic impairment of the articulations of the sequence: the disc, the ligaments, and the facets.

The biopsychosocial concept of low back impairment is in no way refuted by the implementation of the muscular system in the "bio" aspect because the psychosocial manifests itself via muscular actions in anger, fatigue, depression, anxiety, and repetitive stresses. The enigma is starting to be resolved without decreasing the emphasis on the articular aspect, the intervertebral disc, as being responsible for pain and impairment.

REFERENCES

1. Ladin Z. Use of musculoskeletal models in the diagnosis and treatment of low back pain. In: Winters J, Woo SL-O, eds. *Multiple muscle systems: biomechanics and movement organization.* New York: Springer-Verlag, 1990.
2. Lucas D, Bresler B. Stability of ligamentous spine. *Biomechanics Laboratory Report 40,* University of California San Francisco, 1961.
3. De Vries H. *Physiology of exercise,* 3rd ed. Dubuque, Iowa: Wm. C. Brown, 1966:474–476.
4. Marinacci AA. *Applied electromyography.* Philadelphia: Lea & Febiger, 1968:59–61.

5. Gunn CC. *The Gunn approach to the treatment of chronic pain.* Edinburgh: Churchill Livingstone, 1999.
6. Cannon WB, Rosenblueth A. *The supersensitivity of denervated structures.* New York: Macmillan, 1949:1–22, 185.
7. Gunn CC, Milbrandt WE. Tenderness at motor points. *J Bone Joint Surg* 1976;58-A, 6:815–825.
8. Laros GS. Differential diagnosis of low back pain. In: Mayer TG, Mooney V, Gatchel RJ, eds. *Contemporary conservative care for painful spinal disorders.* Philadelphia: Lea & Febiger, 1991:122–130.
9. Mense S. Nociception from skeletal muscle in relation to clinical muscle pain. *Pain* 1993;54:241–289.
10. Edwards RH. Human muscle function and fatigue. *Ciba Found Symp* 1981;82:1–18.
11. Bigland-Ritchie B, Cafarelli A, Vollested NK. Fatigue of submaximal static contractions. *Acta Physiol Scand* 1986;128(Suppl 556):137.
12. Kukulka CG. Human skeletal muscle fatigue. In: Currier DP, Nelson RM, eds. *Contemporary perspectives in rehabilitation.* Philadelphia: FA Davis, 1992.
13. Merton PA. Voluntary strength and fatigue. *J Physiol (London)* 1954; 128:553.
14. Carpenter AF, Georgopoulos AP, Pellizzer G. Motor cortical encoding of serial order in a context-recall task, *Science* 1999;283:1752–1757.
15. McCully K, Faulkner JA. Injury to skeletal muscle fibers of mice following lengthening contractions. *J Appl Physiol* 1985:59:119–126.
16. Newham DJ, Jones DA, Clarkson OM. Repeated high force eccentric exercise in man: effects on muscle pain and damage. *J Appl Physiol* (in press).
17. Aching muscle after exercise. *Lancet* 1987;2:1123–1124.
18. Macdonald AJR. Abnormally tender muscle regions and associated painful movements. *Pain* 1980;8:197–205.
19. Sparto PJ, Parnianpour M, Marras WS, et al. Neuromuscular trunk performance and spinal loading during a fatiguing isometric trunk extension with varying torque requirements. *J Spinal Disord* 1997;10:145–156.
20. Bigland-Ritchie B, Johannson R, Lippold OCJ, et al. Contraction speed and EMG changes during fatigue of sustained maximal voluntary contraction. *J Neurophysiol* 1983;50:313–324.
21. Seidel H, Beyer H, Brauer P. Electromyographic evaluation of back muscle fatigue with repeated sustained contractions of different strengths. *Eur J Appl Physiol* 1987;56:592–602.
22. International Association for the Study of Pain, Subcommittee of toxonomy chronic pain syndromes and definition of pain terms. *Pain* 1986(Suppl); 3:S1.

6. MISCELLANEOUS ABNORMAL CONDITIONS OF THE LOW BACK

Numerous abnormal conditions of the lumbosacral spine, congenital or acquired, may directly cause impairment and discomfort. Some of these are discussed next.

SPONDYLOLYSIS AND SPONDYLOLISTHESIS

Spondylolisthesis became accepted as a low back condition in 1782 (1), when it was mechanically described as a slow displacement of the last lumbar vertebra by Kilian (2). He coined the term *spondylolisthesis*. It was thought that slippage did not occur if the neural arch was intact, until Neurebauer (3) found that it did occur when there was merely a division, a lysis, in the pars interarticularis.

The term *spondylo* relates to the spine, and *lysis* means "dissolution." *Listhesis* is from the Greek word *olisthesis,* meaning "slipping" or "falling." Spondylolisthesis is an anatomic defect of the pars interarticularis that may be unilateral or bilateral. The term also relates to a forward or backward translation subluxation of a superior vertebra upon its immediate inferior vertebra within a functional unit. In the lumbosacral spine the common site of slipping is the fifth vertebra upon the sacrum. Of all reported spondylolisthesis, 70% occurs between L5 and S1; 25%, between L4 and L5; and the remaining 5%, between other lumbar vertebrae (Fig. 6.1).

Shear of a superior upon an inferior vertebra is normally limited by the facets, their capsules, the posterior longitudinal ligament, and the integrity of the annular fibers of the disc. The facets are the predominant factors preventing gliding (Fig. 6.2).

TYPES OF MECHANICAL LISTHESIS

Specific types of listhesis have been postulated (4,5).

Type I: There is an anatomic defect in the pars interarticularis. This is usually seen in adolescents and is considered to be a stress fracture that has healed by fibrous intent and remained stable.

Type II (congenital): The posterior elements are structurally inadequate due to developmental causes.

Type III (degenerative): The facets and their ligaments as supporting structures are degenerated.

Type IV (elongated pedicles): The neural arch is elongated, placing the facets more posteriorly.

Type V (destructive disease): This type of listhesis is a secondary manifestation of a metabolic, metastatic, or infectious disease.

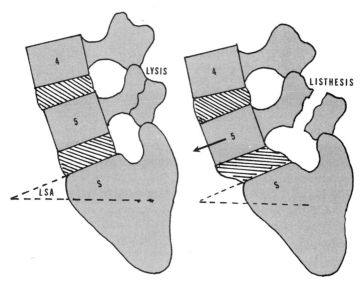

FIG. 6.1. Mechanism of spondylolisthesis. *Left:* The normal alignment of the fifth lumbar vertebra upon the sacrum (S) with an undisplaced lysis of the pars interarticularis of the fifth lumbar vertebra. *Right:* Anterior listhesis of L5 upon the sacrum (LSA) is the lumbosacral angle that shows the potential for downward forward gliding of L5 upon the sacrum.

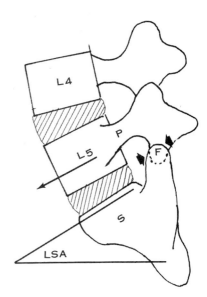

FIG. 6.2. Translation restriction from the facets. The inferior facet (F) of L5 impacts upon the superior facet of S1 to prevent forward sliding upon the sacrum (SD) *(long arrow)* promoted by the angulation of the lumbosacral angle (LSA).

Wiltse (4,5) classified spondylolisthesis as follows:

I. Dysplastic. Congenital abnormality of the upper sacrum or of the arch of the fifth lumbar vertebra.
II. Isthmic. Lesions of the pars interarticularis.
  A. Lytic fatigue.
  B. Elongated but an intact pars interarticularis.
  C. Acute fracture
III. Degenerative. Progressive intersegmental instability.
IV. Traumatic. Fracture or dislocation of the facet joints, allowing forward displacement.
V. Pathologic. Loss of stability secondary to pathologic destruction of the facets or the pars interarticularis.

Type I spondylolisthesis at L5–S1 usually does not progress after 20 years of age until 70 years of age, but listhesis at a higher level tends to progress and invoke neurologic symptoms and signs of spinal stenosis. Lysis may exist and the condition may be symptomatic for the person's entire life. There are situations of a radiologic diagnosis of listhesis with no clinical findings, thus requiring no treatment.

SYMPTOMS OF SPONDYLOLISTHESIS

The major symptom of spondylolisthesis is low back pain frequently radiating into the sacroiliac region but with no dermatomal distribution. Examination reveals a nonspecific limitation of flexibility and often a palpable "ledge" can be felt at the upper edge of the listhesis. Pain is often aggravated by having the patient increase the lumbar lordosis by hyperextending the low back. On rectal examination a mass may be palpable on the anterior aspect of the spine.

Limited straight-leg raising is often found and attributable to tight hamstring muscles. No reason has been found for this condition, as no neurologic abnormalities are found (6,7) causing the limited hamstring muscle elongation.

Treatment

Any treatment will depend upon the severity of the symptoms and the resultant impairment. Taillard (8) found that 6% of the general population has a radiologic defect in a pars interarticularis but without symptoms, whereas 50% of patients with a listhesis do have symptoms (9).

Experimental stress has indicated that fractures can occur from the excessive pressure upon the pars from excessive lumbar lordosis (10,11). Apes, which stand erect without a lumbar lordosis, do not have lysis or spondylolisthesis. Children who ultimately develop lysis or listhesis do not do so until they develop a lumbar lordosis.

Conservative treatment implies improving posture by decreasing lumbar lordosis during the performance of all activities of daily living. This can be assisted by using a brace or a corset that decreases lordosis. This brace (corset) is to be worn until the abdominal muscles are strengthened by exercises and the person can maintain normal posture all day in the performance of daily activities (Fig. 6.3).

Exercises are the mainstay of properly treating spondylolisthesis conservatively (12,13). These exercises must emphasize strengthening the proper abdominal muscles: the deep abdominal obliques, the transversus, and the lumbar multifidus, as will be discussed in Chapter 7 (14–17).

The small intrinsic muscles that attach directly to the vertebra to produce spinal stability are also necessary in treating spondylolisthesis, but the transversus abdominis muscles are the most important, as they stabilize the spine and become activated before any upper-extremity movement is initiated (18–22).

Merely strengthening the trunk muscles without instructing the person in the proper techniques of bending and lifting would be useless; therefore these activities must be taught to the person. The intent is to avoid excessive lordosis during any and all daily activity (Fig. 6.4).

Appropriate surgical procedures have been well documented in the literature (23,24) and are beyond the scope of this text. The decision to resort to surgery depends on the symptoms and the degree and type of listhesis, which is a radiologic measurement.

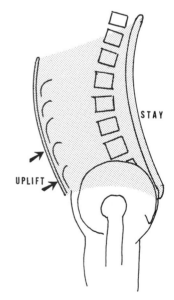

STAY

UPLIFT

FIG. 6.3. Concepts of low back bracing. A brace intended to decrease lordosis must have an inflexible reinforcement—stays—posteriorly that conforms to the desired curvature. The upper contact of these stays is at T12 vertebra, and the lower aspect is at the sacrum. The anterior portion of the brace (corset) must also have an uplift of the lower abdominal wall.

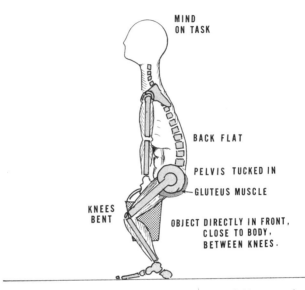

FIG. 6.4. Proper lifting technique. All aspects of proper lifting are shown in this illustration.

SPINAL STENOSIS

Spinal stenosis has been defined as a condition of any type of narrowing of the spinal canal, the nerve root canals, or the vertebral foramina. Narrowing of the spinal canal involves not only the reduced anterior–posterior and lateral diameters of the canal, but also the cross-sectional configuration of the canal. This narrowing can be congenital or acquired, from disc herniation or facet hypertrophy. Clinical symptoms indicate the need for exact radiologic measurement in which an anterior–posterior width of less than 10 mm is considered pathologic (25) (Fig. 6.5).

The clinical syndrome of spinal stenosis is subjective, is often vague, and may even lack substantiation from a clinical examination. Back pain is the most frequent complaint, with nerve root entrapment coming later and being less acute than the symptoms from a disc herniation into the foramen.

The initial leg symptoms are usually feelings of coldness, tingling or burning, or of the legs falling asleep. There may be symptoms of early-morning "stiffness" that improve with activity. Back pain is more pronounced after prolonged standing or after a period of walk

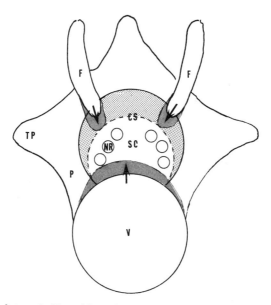

FIG. 6.5. Spinal stenosis. Viewed from above, a spinal segment contains the vertebra (V), pedicle (P), transverse process (TP), and spinal canal (SC). In congenital stenosis (CS) the canal is anatomically narrowed by osseous tissue. Hypertrophied facets (F) contribute. Narrowing occurs from posterior herniation of the disc or osteophytes (*arrow*). The nerve roots (NR) can be encroached upon.

ing. It is felt less from reclining, especially in the side-lying position with the knees and hips flexed, the so-called fetal position.

With progression of the syndrome, symptoms of neurogenic claudication appear, which are the classic signs and symptoms of the syndrome. These symptoms are leg pain, termed *cramping,* after a progressively limited period of walking similar to the symptoms of vascular claudication. With progression of limited walking due to pain, motor signs of weakness develop.

Contrary to vascular claudication, relief of symptoms occurs not only from cessation of walking but from assumption of a flexed posture, which anatomically lengthens the spinal canal. After a period of assuming this posture, walking is again possible, albeit for a limited distance and duration. As compared with vascular claudication, the distal extremity pulses are palpable and full.

Treatment of spinal stenosis is to decrease the lumbar lordosis, as was indicated in the treatment of spondylolisthesis, and by the same means: exercise, corset, brace, and ergonomic training. When the neurologic findings appear and progress with objective neurologic deficits, surgical intervention is indicated. This indicates decompression with or without fusion to maintain stability.

SCOLIOSIS

Idiopathic juvenile scoliosis is usually asymptomatic and is cosmetic with psychologic sequelae. It is only when adult scoliosis appears, after closure of the epiphyses, that, depending upon the severity of the scoliosis, degenerative changes occur that progress and become symptomatic.

The anatomic abnormalities that occur during the progress of scoliosis, for which a cause is still not understood, involve the vertebrae becoming wedged during maturation, which is also true of the discs (Fig. 6.6). The vertebrae also rotate and form lateral curva-

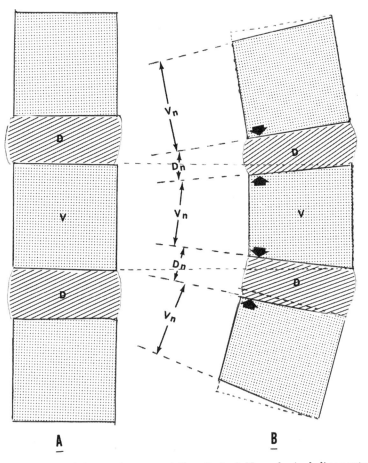

FIG. 6.6. Segmental changes in severe adult scoliosis. **A:** Normal spinal alignment vertebra (V) and discs (D). **B:** Lateral curvature in scoliosis, with the vertebra narrow on the concave side of the curve (Vn) and with the disc narrow on the concave side (Dn) from unequal pressure (*arrows*).

tures, further causing damage of the discs and the vert
These changes are characteristic of discogenic disease
facet irregularities posteriorly (Fig. 6.7).

These degenerative changes are more prominent and progressive
if the curves are not in the center of gravity alignment (Fig. 6.8).

These structural changes of the vertebrae, the discs, and the facets
lead to inflexibility, weight-bearing pain, and functional impairment
with pain on movement and the performance of activities of daily
living.

Treatment is conservative management, as discussed in the treatment of low back pain (Chapter 7), with surgery as a last alternative.

PIRIFORMIS SYNDROME

The role of the piriformis muscle producing the classic symptoms and
signs of sciatica was initially proposed by Yeoman in 1928 (26), when
he postulated that the proximity of the sciatic nerve to the piriformis
muscle could account for compression of the nerve (Fig. 6.9) when the
muscle contracts or is shortened for any reason (27,28). Surgical release of the piriformis muscle has confirmed this compression (29).

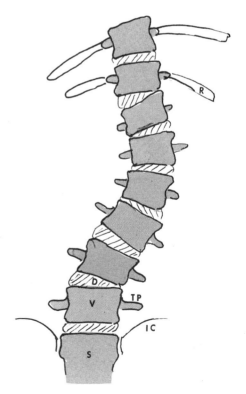

FIG. 6.7. Structural changes in the lumbar spine of scoliosis. In severe adult scoliosis there is segmental rotation and lateral flexion with vertebral body and intervertebral disc changes. There are abnormal changes of the ribs that deform the thoracic cage. D, disc; IC, iliac crest; R, ribs; S, sacrum; TP, transverse process; V, vertebra.

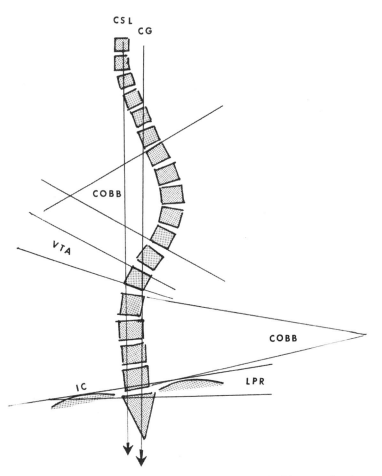

FIG. 6.8. Scoliosis alignment with the center of gravity. A double curve, lumbar and thoracic, as depicted with Cobb measurements depicts vertebral changes (VTA) with compression on the concave side of the curve. Here the spine is not aligned with the center of gravity (CG), causing more vertebral compressive stress. The iliac crest (IC) indicates a change in the lumbar–vertebral relationship (LPR). In this case there is elevation of the right iliac crest, indicating pelvic obliquity.

The clinical syndrome is suggested by the following:

1. A history of local trauma
2. Pain and local tenderness over the greater sciatic notch and/or the piriformis muscle area
3. A palpable spindle or sausage mass at the anatomic location of the piriformis muscle
4. Reproduction of the sciatic pain distribution by straight-leg raising with simultaneous active or passive internal rotation of the femur

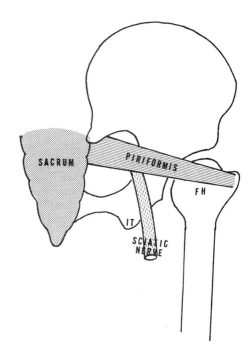

FIG. 6.9. The piriformis muscle. The piriformis muscle and its anatomic proximity of the sciatic nerve are shown. The muscle attaches to the tuberosity of the femoral head (FH). It is an external rotator of the femur and compresses the nerve against the ischial tuberosity (IT) when it contracts.

5. Reproduction of the sciatic pain distribution from percutaneous pressure applied to the piriformis muscle externally or vaginally
6. Relief of pain upon infusion of 1% lidocaine into the piriformis muscle
7. Failure to identify other pathology of the lumbosacral spine on CT scanning or MRI studies
8. Confirmation of the syndrome electromyographically (30)

Clinically, the piriformis syndrome can be diagnosed by placing the patient into the classic position termed by Fishman et al. (31) as FAIR (by placing the hip in flexion, adduction, and internal rotation) (Fig. 6.10).

Electromyographic confirmation (31) is done measuring the peroneal H-reflex (32,33). While the patient is in the anatomic position a program such as the following (31) is used.

1. Ultrasound 2.0 to 2.5 W/cm^2 over the piriformis area for 10 to 15 minutes
2. Hot pack over the area for 10 minutes
3. Stretch the piriformis muscle in the manner used diagnostically

If there is not significant and permanent benefit, surgical resection of the piriformis muscle can be advocated.

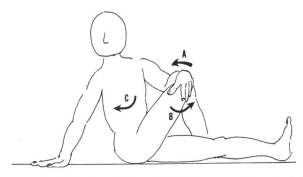

FIG. 6.10. FAIR: the piriformis position test. With the normal leg extended, the other leg is flexed at the hip, adducted, then rotated internally. That stretches the piriformis muscle and compresses the nerve.

SACROILIAC DISEASE

In 1905 Goldthwait and Osgood (34) introduced a condition that they termed *sacroiliac strain,* but Bourdillon in 1970 stated, "The range of motion of the sacro-iliac joint is so small and demonstration [of disease] by direct palpation is both difficult and unconvincing . . . indeed the existence and importance of sacro-iliac mobility is still a subject of argument" (35). This argument persists today in many minds.

The sacro-iliac joint is an extremely stable joint by virtue of its numerous incongruous joint surfaces and its powerful anterior and posterior ligaments. Unless there is clear radiologic evidence of subluxation or dislocation, the clinical diagnosis of sacroiliac pathology remains questioned. Mooney (36) has stated, "It is difficult to separate pain emerging from the sacro-iliac joint from pain radiating from the facet joints because there is overlapping innervation."

Degenerative changes are noted in the sacro-iliac joints in 67% of persons 55 years of age, implying that some movement of these joints must have occurred, although those studied were asymptomatic (37,38).

In studying a person to elicit the possibility of a sacro-iliac joint disorder, the joint must be passively moved and the symptoms elicited from that movement.

This passive movement is to place the patient supine on the examining table and have the examiner push down firmly on both anterior–superior iliac spines simultaneously and alternately. With the patient lying on his or her side, the pelvis is directly pressed down.

Injection of an analgesic agent into the joint with relief of the pain is also diagnostic and therapeutic.

Treatment

Treatment of the patient who has a confirmed diagnosis of sacroiliac pathology as the source of the pain is by applying a tight-fitting girdle and injections of analgesics and steroids into the joint. Surgical fusion may be needed.

SACRO-ILIAC PATHOLOGY SECONDARY TO A PELVIC FRACTURE

A pelvic fracture may cause secondary sacro-iliac deformity with resultant pain in that joint. A pelvic fracture may cause disruption of the pelvic ring at the symphysis pubis and the sacro-iliac joint(s). When a patient has sustained a pelvic fracture anywhere in the pelvis, radiologic evaluation of the entire ring is mandated to ascertain the integrity of the sacro-iliac joints so that appropriate treatment can be initiated early (Fig. 6.11).

SACRALIZATION OF A TRANSVERSE PROCESS

A transverse process of the fifth lumbar vertebra may be congenitally elongated, allowing its distal tip to fuse with the medial aspect of the ileum, resulting in a pseudoarthrosis. This may be noted radiologically and may be asymptomatic but may cause symptoms by its restricting movement of the fifth lumbar vertebra, which causes disc degeneration from excessive movement of either adjacent vertebra. Local pain may occur from movement of the fifth vertebra, and when the pseudoarthrosis is noted an injection of an analgesic agent will confirm that the false joint is the cause of mechanical low back pain. Recurrence of the symptoms may require surgical intervention to resect the pseudoarthrosis.

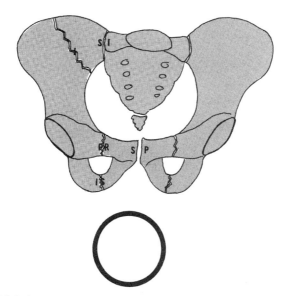

FIG. 6.11. Pelvic fractures. The pelvic "ring" is shown with fractures of the ileum (I), pelvic ramus (PR) ischial spine (IS), and with separation of the symphysis pubis (SP).

REFERENCES

1. Herbiniaux G. *Traité sur divers accouchements laborieux et sur les polypes de la matrice.* Brussels, Belgium: JL DeBoubers, 1782.
2. Kilian HF. *Schilderungen neuer Beckenformen and ihres Verhaltens im Leben.* Mannheim, Germany: Verlag von Bassermann & Mathy, 1854.
3. Neugebauer FL. Die Entstehung der Spondylolistehsis. *Zetralblatt fur Gynakologie* 1881;53:264.
4. Wiltse LL, Winter RB. Terminology and measurement of spondylolis-thesis. *J Bone Joint Surg* 1983;65A:768.
5. Wiltse LL, Newman PH, MacNab I. Classification of spondylolisthesis. *Clin Orthop* 1976;17:23.
6. Barash HL, Galante JO, Lambert CN, et al. Spondylolisthesis and tight hamstrings. *J Bone Joint Surg* 1970;52:1319–1328.
7. Phalen GS, Dickson JA. Spondylolisthesis and tight hamstrings. *J Bone Joint Surg* 1956;38A:946.
8. Taillard WF. Etiology of spondylolisthesis. *Clin Orthop* 1976;117:30–39.
9. Magora A. Conservative treatment in spondylolisthesis. *Clin Orthop* 1976;117:74–79.
10. Eisenstein S. Spondylolysis: a skeletal investigation of two population groups. *J Bone Joint Surg (Br)* 1978;60:488–494.
11. Troup JDG. Mechanical factors in spondylolisthesis and spondylolysis. *Clin Orthop* 1976;117:59–67.
12. O'Sullivan PB, Phyty GDM, Twomey LT, et al. Evaluation of specific sta-bilizing exercise in the treatment of chronic low back pain with radio-logical diagnosis of spondylolysis or spondylolisthesis. *Spine* 1997;22: 24:2959..
13. Bergmark S. Stability of the lumbar spine: a study in mechanical engi-neering. *Acta Orthop Scand* 1989;230(Suppl 60):20–24.
14. Goel V, Kong W, Han J, et al. A combined finite element and optimizing investigation of lumbar spine mechanics with and without muscles. *Spine* 1993:18:1531–1541.
15. Kaigle A, Holm S, Hansson R. Experimental instability in the lumbar spine. *Spine* 1995;20:421–430.
16. Panjabi M, Abumi K, Duranceau J, et al. Spinal stability and interseg-mental muscles forces: a biomechanical model. *Spine* 1989:14:194–199.
17. Wilke H, Wolf S, Claes LE, et al. Stability increase of the lumbar spine with different muscle groups. *Spine* 1995:20:192–198.
18. Gardner-Morse M, Stokes I, Laible J. Role of muscles in lumbar spine stability in maximum extension efforts. *J Orthop Res* 1995:13:802–808.
19. Cholewicke J, McGill S. Mechanical stability of the in vivo lumbar spine: implications for injury and chronic low back pain. *Clin Biomech* 1996: 11:1–15.
20. Zetterberg C, Andersson GB, Schultz AB. The activity of individual trunk muscles during heavy lifting. *Spine* 1987:12:1035–1040.
21. Hodges P, Richardson C. Feedforward contraction of transversus abdo-minis is not influenced by the direction of arm movement. *Exp Brain Res* 1997:114:362–370.
22. Hodges P, Richardson C. Inefficient muscular stabilization of the lum-bar spine associated with low back pain: a motor control evaluation of transversus abdominis. *Spine* 1996;21:2640–2650.
23. Hensinger N, Lang JR, MacEwen GD. Surgical management of spondy-lolisthesis in children and adolescents. *Spine* 1976;1:207–216.

24. Savastano AA, Novoch J. Review of the conservative and operative management of spondylolisthesis in the lumbosacral spine. *Int Surg* 1972; 57:571–576.

25. Huizinga J, Heiden JA, Vinken PJ. The human lumbar vertebral canal: a biometric study. *Proc R Acad Sci* (Amsterdam) 1952;C55:22.

26. Yeoman W. The relation of arthritis of the sacro-iliac joint to sciatica with an analysis of 100 cases. *Lancet* 1928;2:1177–1180.

27. Frieberg AH. Sciatic pain and its relief by operations on muscle and fascia. *Arch Surg* 1937;34:337–350.

28. Thiele GH. Coccygodynia and pain in the superior gluteal region and down the back of the thigh. *JAMA* 1937;101:1271–1275.

29. Durrani A, Winnie AP. Piriformis syndrome: an underdiagnosed cause of sciatica. *J Pain Symptom Manage* 1991;6:374–371.

30. Fishman LM, Zybert PA. Electrophysiological evidence of piriformis syndrome. *Arch Phys Med Rehabil* 1992;73:351–364.

31. Fishman LM, Dombi GW, Michaelsen C, et al. Piriformis syndrome: diagnosis, treatment and outcome—a 10-year study. *Arch Phys Med Rehabil* 2002;83:295–301.

32. Hugan M. Methodology of the Hoffmann reflex in man. In: Desmedt JE, ed. *New developments in electromyography and chemical neurophysiology,* vol. 3, Basel: Karger, 1973:227–293.

33. Braddom RI, Johnson EW. Standardization of H reflex and diagnostic use in S1 radiculopathy. *Arch Phys Med Rehabil* 1974:55:161–166.

34. Goldthwait JE, Osgood RB. *A consideration of the pelvic articulation from an anatomical, pathological and clinical standpoint.* Boston: M & SJ, 1905;152:593.

35. Bourdillon JF. *Spinal manipulation.* New York: Appleton-Century-Crofts, 1970.

36. Don Tigney RL. Function and pathomechanics of the sacroiliac joints: a review. *Phys Ther* 1985;65:35.

37. Mooney V. The subacute patient: to operate or not? This is a good question. In: Mayer TG, Mooney V, Gatchel RJ, eds. *Contemporary conservative care for painful spinal disorders.* Philadelphia: Lea & Febiger, 1991.

38. Walheim GG, Selvik G. Mobility of the pubic symphysis: In vivo measurements with an electromechanic method and a roentgen stereophotogrammetric method. *Clin Orthop* 1984;191:129–135.

7. TREATMENT PROTOCOLS FOR LOW BACK DISORDERS

The term *pain,* not *impairment,* is considered of the greatest concern to the patient. The International Association for the Study of Pain (IASP) Committee on Taxonomy defined *pain* as "an unpleasant sensory and emotional experience associated with actual or potential tissue damage, or described in terms of such damage." "Pain is always subjective. Each individual learns the application of the word through experiences related to injury in early life" (1–4).

This definition implies that pain is experienced only within the context of adult human consciousness and imposes on all others the impossible task of proving their experience without access to the means by which pain can be proven (5).

Anand et al. (6) charged that this definition of a "verbal self report is scientifically unreasonable." This may be particularly true in patients with pain in the low back when there usually is not a discernible etiology. This is even more true when acute pain becomes chronic pain in spite of what has been considered "appropriate treatment."

Pain is considered to be present when there are "pain behaviors" or when there is the symptom of pain as expressed by the patient. Nonspecific low back pain has been defined as an "unresolved medical condition" after 6 weeks of treatment (7). This definition reveals professional skepticism but is what I define as an enigma, because no one apparently knows the cause(s) of chronic low back pain (8,9).

Acute pain is commonly defined as the "normal predicted physiological response to an adverse chemical, thermal or mechanical stimulus . . . associated with surgery, trauma or acute illness" (10). Neuronal sensitization leading to pain occurs within 20 minutes of injury and can initiate histologic changes leading to long-term behavioral changes within a day. Acute pain should therefore be viewed as the initiation phase of an extensive, persistent nociceptive and behavioral cascade lasting for a span of time. Early minimization of pain can improve outcomes.

Cascades of Acute Pain*

Stimulus
↓
Neurotransmitter release (glutamate, asparate, enkephalin, neuropeptide, substance P, gene-related peptide)

*Modified after Carr DB, Goudal LC (10).

↓

Electrophysiologic response (excitatory postsynaptic potential, sensitization)

↓

Intracellular response (calcium, nitric oxide, protein kinase C, etc.)

↓

Neural structural response (spouting, remodeling, cell death)

↓

Neurophysiologic responses (perception, aversion, avoidance, suffering, chronic pain syndrome)

↓

Quality of life

In evaluating all treatment modalities in the treatment of chronic pain it can be concluded that "no single therapeutic intervention has been demonstrated to be effective in the treatment of chronic low back pain." Why a certain patient becomes chronically painful in spite of standard treatment remains a major source of study (11).

Treatment of acute pain must identify the particular subgroup that may become chronic (12–16). An aspect of evaluating the efficacy of any treatment protocol is whether the pain is acute, chronic, or recurrent. Factors relating to the duration of pain must be ascertained before a condition can be termed chronic. Besides regarding subjective pain, restoration of function must be documented and be the basis of benefit from any treatment (17).

Pain mechanisms have been thoroughly discussed in the literature (18), and pain neurologic mechanisms and psychological aspects are undergoing rapid evaluation. The current neurophysiologic aspect of pain asserts that from the "injured tissue" C and A alpha fibers convey nociceptive impulses to the dorsal horn of the spinal cord. Impulses then cross the cord to ascend via spinothalamic tracts to the hypothalamus, limbic system, and the thalamus to the cerebral cortex, where pain is recognized. The dorsal horn integrates incoming signals (19,20).

In 1965 Melzack-Wall postulated a gate control theory that emphasized the mechanisms in the central nervous system that control the perception of a noxious stimulus (21,22). This theory did not incorporate the long-term changes in the central nervous system initiated by the noxious input with other external factors that impress upon the individual (23) (Fig. 7.1). The noxious effects of neurologic transmission are usually transient and exist only during the initial period of healing. Huge nociceptive input, however, can permanently change spinal cord function through excitatory effects of amino acids (24). The plasticity of the central nervous system, especially at the level of the brain, occurs because synaptic potentiation is altered by repetitive noxious

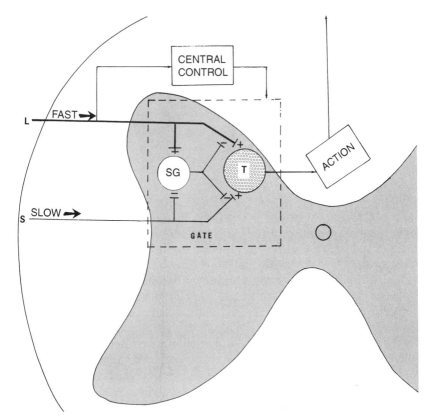

FIG. 7.1. The gate theory of Wall-Melzack. The fast impulses (L) transmitted via unmyelinated nerves enter the gray matter of the spinal cord into the substantia gelatinosum (SG) (Rexed layers I and II) on their way to the lateral spinal thalamic tracts. (−) indicate a blocking of the impulses from upper systems and (+) unrestricted passage.

stimuli (25,26). This plasticity and ultimate newer or modified "neural connections" explain how the brain can generate "pain" in the absence of input from peripheral nociceptors. Phantom limb pain or pain in neurologic paraplegics is an example (27) (Fig. 7.2).

Pain behaviors can be generated, or perpetuated, by previous conditioned cues of the environment or by the expectation of pain and suffering. Injury not only produces pain but also leads to stress, resulting in neural, hormonal, and behavioral activities.

The sensory awareness of tissue trauma represents information crucial for adaptation and survival. Most of the time it serves us well, but when it persists it contributes to disability and suffering (28). Suffering and pain are distinct phenomena and are not synonymous. Not all pain causes suffering and not all suffering is expressed as

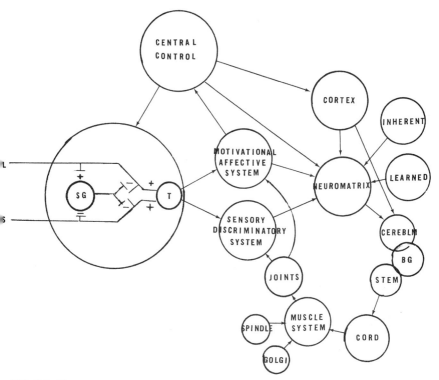

FIG. 7.2. Neuromatrix concept of Melzack. On the left is the concept of the gate system affecting pain perception. The fibers labeled L are the large fibers; those labeled S are the small fibers that project to the substanita gelatinosum (SG) in the gray matter of the cord. These impulses project to the (T) cells. The − indicates inhibitory; + is excitatory. Beyond the gate exists a neuromatrix between the cortex and the thalamus and limbic system that contains inherent patterns modified by experience.

pain. Suffering connotes enduring something unpleasant, dealing with something inconvenient, experiencing a disability, and having a feeling of helplessness.

Of the extraneous factors that affect pain, fear of the significance of the pain or of recurrence also has an effect upon the musculature of the spine, which is a contributing factor to the impairment and pain (Fig. 7.3). The emotions are therefore "extraneous" contributors to impaired neuromuscular function. For more than 40 years the limbic system has predominated as the dominant site in the brain where emotions exist. but the limbic system may be bypassed in recognizing pain in the cortex, as the nociceptive impulses are instantaneously transmitted through the amygdala (Figs. 7.4 and 7.5) (28,29).

(text continues on page 110)

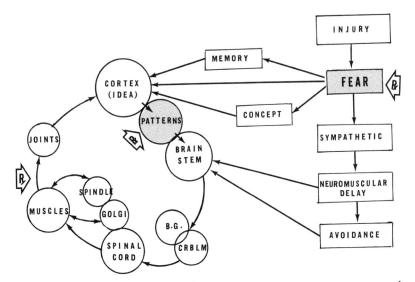

FIG. 7.3. Neurophysiologic effect of fear. The effect of fear upon the neuromuscular system is depicted.

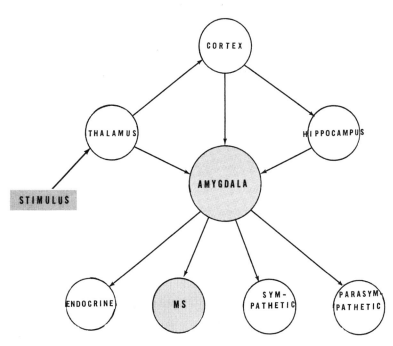

FIG. 7.4. Information flow to and from the amygdala. The amygdala has numerous connections within the brain system. As information (stimulus) arrives from the periphery it is transmitted as a sensory input to the thalamus, then to the cortex, from which there is flow to the hippocampus and the amygdala. The afferents from the amygdala flow to the endocrine system and to the sympathetic, parasympathetic, and musculoskeletal systems.

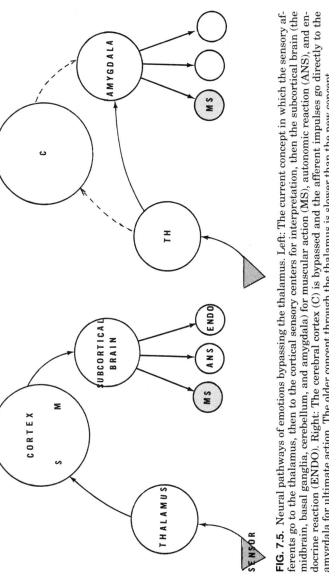

FIG. 7.5. Neural pathways of emotions bypassing the thalamus. Left: The current concept in which the sensory afferents go to the thalamus, then to the cortical sensory centers for interpretation, then the subcortical brain (the midbrain, basal ganglia, cerebellum, and amygdala) for muscular action (MS), autonomic reaction (ANS), and endocrine reaction (ENDO). Right: The cerebral cortex (C) is bypassed and the afferent impulses go directly to the amygdala for ultimate action. The older concept through the thalamus is slower than the new concept.

All these factors indicate that nociception, acute and severe, may leave a permanent neurologic change in the central nervous system and act instantaneously, and that "extraneous" factors such as fear may intensify the reaction. All these factors, and many others, must be evaluated as they influence treatment protocols.

MANAGEMENT OF ACUTE SYMPTOMS OF LOW BACK DISORDERS

Because neuronal sensitization and remodeling of the central nervous system occurs within 20 minutes of injury, initiating the "cascade of pain," early intervention is indicated. The benefit of acute intervention is the relief of subjective discomfort, anxiety, apprehension, or fear of permanent disability.

As was implied early in this text, the impression of low back pain and impairment as being "an incurable and irreversible disease" must be immediately addressed with the patient. The concept of disease must be dispelled with an explanation that the condition is essentially a temporary, albeit acute, disruption of the normal mechanics of the spine from an inadvertent movement.

Each of the symptoms must be clarified as to the tissue site and the mechanics whereby these tissue have been "injured," and the term *injured* must be compared to an ankle sprain or similar soft-tissue insult that has a limited duration and usually no persistent impairment.

Fear of permanence and even more important recurrence must be addressed early. Pain must also be addressed as being a sign of insult but not a sinister omen, and as an indication of tissue injury that will abate with time and appropriate medication and modalities. Function must be restored early and without further tissue damage.

Fear is eliminated and active participation of the patient is ensured by this early explanation. It must be remembered that in an acute and painful disabling situation the physician literally becomes a savior in whose hands the future of the patient resides. All patients must be considered as knowledgeable and able to understand a meaningful explanation. Terms such as *disc disease, degenerative arthritis,* and *spasms* must be avoided or at best used but carefully explained.

Any medication must also be explained as to purpose, indication, duration, and possible side effects. The reason usually is for temporary relief of pain to permit "normal healing of the injured tissues." Such an explanation regarding modalities must be clarified as being adjunctive and not curative, but merely to "hasten normal tissue recovery."

Total recovery of function must be the goal and not merely total and immediate relief of pain, as pain may persist, albeit with diminution, as function is restored. The restoration of function must be stressed; basically, this is the major concern of all patients. Loss of activities of daily function resides in the mind of the patient, although that is not necessarily expressed in the patient's history.

Addressing Acute Pain

As in any neuromuscular impairment, elimination or diminution of acute pain may involve the use of oral analgesics, as well as many other modalities. These measures are not specific but are used merely to diminish pain that prevents daily function. The usual medications are the nonsteroidal antiinflammatory drugs (NSAIDs) or acetaminophen, which inhibit cyclooxygenase in both the spinal cord and the periphery, thus diminishing hyperalgesia at those neural levels (30).

Opioid analgesics, which reduce inflammation, are the basis for relief of moderate to severe pain occurring from injured tissues. They act on the dorsal horn of the spinal cord, where they impede transmission of nociceptive impulses (31). Opioids can be administered in numerous ways: orally, intramuscularly, subcutaneously, intravenously, and even rectally. Combinations of systemic opioids and NSAIDs are widely used and effective.

STEROIDS AND NONSTEROIDAL MEDICATIONS

When nonsteroidal medication is ineffective or the pain is too severe, steroids may be utilized. All the side effects of nausea, gastric irritation, and so on, must be understood, and when side effects occur, the drug must be stopped. These medications should be used only over the short term because prolonged use inevitably causes undesirable side effects.

If steroids given orally are beneficial, this may suffice, but if pain recurs or fails to be significantly improved, opiates given intramuscularly or epidurally may be indicated (32).

Epidural Steroids

The epidural approach of injecting steroids is through a spinal needle entering the epidural space. The technique involves inserting a spinal needle in the desired spinal level and between two palpable posterior spinal processes. As the needle passes the longitudinal ligament, it enters the epidural space, where there is negative pressure; the plunger is then pulled toward the needle. If the needle has been inserted past the epidural space, it enters the dural space that contains spinal fluid. As this fluid is under pressure the plunger is pushed back and fluid enters the syringe. Injecting the steroid at this point would be an intradural injection, if that is what is indicated (Fig. 7.6).

Besides nonsteroidal antiinflammatory medications, other medications have been advocated. Most low back disorders incur protective muscular spasm. A sustained muscular contraction prevents motion of the injured spine and may be a site of nociception. This muscular spasm must be addressed. This involves the use of numerous modalities.

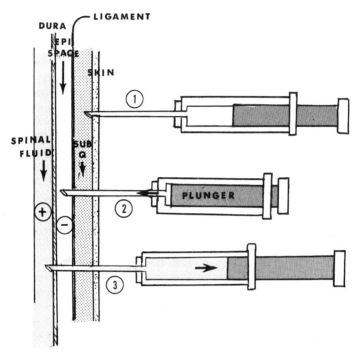

FIG. 7.6. Technique for epidural injection. Entering in the midline at the desired spinal level after penetrating the skin, the subcutaneous tissue (SUB Q), the posterior longitudinal ligament is met and also penetrated. Further penetration enters the epidural space, where there is negative pressure (−) and no fluid. That is the space where the steroids are injected. Further penetration would enter the spinal fluid where there is pressure (+) that enters the syringe and ejects the plunger.

Numerous oral medications have their proponents, but most are ineffective and have undesirable side effects. To decrease this muscular component of acute low back disorders other modalities are more effective than medications, although both can be used simultaneously.

PHYSICAL MODALITIES FOR TREATMENT OF LOW BACK PAIN
Most of the treatment modalities can be considered as placebos if the definition of *placebo* (33) is (Latin): "shall please: an inactive substance given to satisfy patient's demand for medicine." In the case of low back disorders a therapeutic modality can replace an inactive substance.

Bed Rest
For centuries bed rest has been advocated in treating acute low back pain, and it can be considered beneficial in the initial phase. Bed rest for a few days in severe acute low back pain, used with other modalities and medications, is acceptable but longer than 2 or 3 days is

contraindicated as disuse results in atrophy, psychologic depen-
dence, and chronicity.

Cryotherapy

For centuries cryotherapy—the local application of cold over an
acute, painful musculoskeletal injury—has been accepted as beneficial for the relief of pain and the diminution of the sequelae of tissue
injury. Three mechanisms of its physiologic effect have been postulated: (a) the adaptation of pain receptors, (b) a counterirritant effect,
and (c) a neurogenic effect (34–36). The local application of cold decreases bleeding and thus the release of platelets, and decreases local
tissue metabolism, which produces algogens and neutralizes local his-
tamine formation. Ice decreases edema, decreases local muscle spasm
by decreasing the sensitivity of the muscle spindle system, and elevates the threshold of pain-transmitting impulses. Ice is a valuable
modality in the presence of pain and impairment but is also a valuable
adjunct to such modalities as exercise. Local cold may be administered
by ice cubes in a plastic bag applied to the low back for 20 minutes and
repeated four times daily for 3 or 4 days, then followed by the application of heat. Besides minimizing the acute pain and inflammation, its
major benefit is that it permits active motion by the patient and can be
applied at home, where exercises are performed.

Therapeutic Heat

The therapeutic benefit of applying local heat is vascular dilatation,
which alters metabolic activity, hemodynamic function, neural response, and modification of collagen tissue (37–39). Heating an area
over a peripheral nerve induces analgesia distal to the application
site, in the dermatomal area. Metabolic rate increases two- to three-
fold with every 10°C rise. Superficial heat causes a reflex post-
ganglionic sympathetic nerve activity to the smooth muscles of
the blood vessels, thereby supplying more blood flow to the deeper
organs, especially the muscles.

Heat is indicated after a brief period of cryotherapy to bring blood
supply to the area and facilitate healing. Local heat can be applied
with hot moist packs, ultrasound, or infrared equipment. Care must
be taken that heat not be applied over an area that is insensitive because of a neurologic disease such as diabetes and peripheral neuropathy. The duration of an application is usually 20 minutes several
times a day for 3 to 5 days. It has specific value when it is used to pre-
cede exercise, which is its major benefit. Again this modality can be
applied at home before or after an exercise program or even without
exercise as the pain demands.

Ultrasound heat is considered effective, as its penetration is
deeper than moist heat, but its efficacy is diminished because it

must be administered in a therapy department, which requires travel and time constraints, even when it is accompanied by other modalities (39).

Manipulation

Chiropractic treatment has been considered to be as effective as standard physical therapy, although at this time no scientific basis has been discovered for its efficacy. Chiropractic therapy traces its origin to 1895, when Daniel David Palmer treated and helped a deaf janitor by spinal manipulation. He postulated that many, if not most, medical problems were due to spinal misalignments. This could certainly be true in lumbar spine pathology (40,41), but as yet this view has not been confirmed by objective study.

The benefits of manipulation have been postulated to occur from the following:

1. Mobilization of a facet (zygapophyseal) joint that has been entrapped from an inadvertent movement
2. Release of an entrapped meniscus in a facet joint that has occurred from an inappropriate motion
3. Release of entrapped synovial capsule within the facet joint
4. Restoration of the mechanism of the mechanoreceptors of a joint
5. Effect upon the spindle and Golgi apparatus from an abrupt motion incurred by the manipulation, thus releasing the muscular contraction that immobilizes the joint
6. Psychologic effect of the laying on of hands and experiencing audible sounds (snap) of the manipulation

Manipulation may be harmful when there is severe structural instability of the vertebral units being treated or if there is infection or malignancy present. These contraindications to manipulation have been postulated by national chiropractic standards.

Manipulation differs from mobilization in that in the former the force is abrupt but in the latter is gradual. The end result is to free the joint into a physiologic position and "realign" what has been misaligned by the detrimental forces causing pathology.

The value of manipulation remains to be confirmed by controlled radiologic studies. Currently, the benefit is subjective in acute cases, albeit beneficial, but the frequency of manipulation and its indications remain mute and the long-term benefit remains unconfirmed.

Traction

Traction has been used since the time of Hippocrates yet today remains unconfirmed as to lasting value in treating mechanical low back pain. It was felt that distraction of the spine retracted the herniating disc, but this has not been confirmed (42–44).

Traction does distract the intervertebral disc spaces, but its main effect appears to be to decrease the lumbar lordosis, which

1. Opens the intervertebral foramen.
2. Separates the facets.
3. Elongates the erector spinae muscles.
4. "Stiffens" the annular fibers of the intervertebral discs, thus unloading the internal pressure within the nucleus.
5. Decreases the length of the nerve roots and their dura, thereby decreasing the tension upon the roots.

As stated, its direct effect upon the bulge of a disc has not been confirmed.

Although the objective benefit of traction has yet to be proven, the various types of traction need to be enumerated and their application described. Autotraction, which is self-applied traction, has been advocated. Its direct effect upon the bulge of a disc has not been confirmed, but if it gives benefit it can be applied at home as frequently as desired and is beneficial. Numerous types of traction have been expounded in the literature, but they will not be discussed here.

EXERCISE IN THE TREATMENT OF LOW BACK DISORDERS TO REGAIN SPINAL STABILITY

Previous chapters have noted that the human osteoligamentous lumbar spine is not stable and buckles in the neutral posture under compressive loads of approximately 90 N, which is significantly less than the body weight of the upper torso. The muscular system supplies the needed support to protect the articular structures—the discs and the facets—and prevents unwanted joint displacement.

Recruitment of Muscles in Spinal Stability

Normal trunk muscle function requires the recruitment of specific trunk muscle groups before an anticipated activity needed for a specific activity. Failure to ensure spinal stability before committing spinal muscles to the required task is a major source of low back impairment and pain. Not having the strength and endurance of these recruitment muscles makes subsequent contraction of activation muscles inappropriate.

Spinal stability is accomplished by incurring what has been called *muscle stiffness,* implying co-contraction of the agonist and antagonists muscles (flexors and extensors) about that joint. Resultant joint stiffness occurs even if the muscle contraction is minimal. Twenty-five percent of maximum voluntary contraction has been shown to provide maximum joint stiffness.

Co-contraction of antagonist trunk muscles acts to stiffen the erect spine. In the neutral position these muscles must adequately

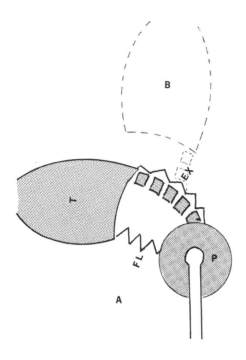

FIG. 7.7. Trunk flexor-extensor coactivation. **A:** The erect, stiff spine in the neutral position made so by the guywire support of antagonist muscle groups. The lumbar spine supports the trunk (T) and head (H). In the neutral position the muscles are contracting minimally and the spine is vulnerable to injury when the supported trunk moves the slightest. **B:** Flexion in which the flexors contract appropriately and the extensors relax proportionately. All this muscular activity is guided by spindle system–Golgi intervention. (Modified from Cholewichi J, Panjabi MM, Khachatryan. Stabilizing function of trunk flexor–extensor muscles around a neutral spine posture. *Spine* 1997;22:2207–2212.)

co-contract at the appropriate time and with proper strength (Fig. 7.7) (45–49).

Because appropriate muscular strength, endurance, and coordination are necessary for proper spinal function, specific exercises are necessary. Before evaluating the efficacy of any treatment modality the question always arises, "Why does acute back pain become chronic?" (50). Jayson postulates that chronic pain is not the same as acute pain that lasts longer but feels that there is increasing evidence that vascular damage and central neuromodulation are fundamental in the development of chronic low back pain syndromes. If that is true all modalities must address this concept; exercise does so in many ways.

A great many cases of low back pain, especially when accompanied by leg radiation, are due to disc herniations. The cause of pain remains unclear but currently is considered to be more chemical than mechanical (51). A disc herniation usually resolves (resorbs) and is considered to be absorbed by vascular invasion (52). How any or most of the treatment modalities favorably affect these changes remains to be determined.

For many years exercise has been the major conservative modality in the treatment of low back pain—either acute, chronic, or recurrent—and with or without leg radiation. Which specific exercise(s) is appropriate and proven to be effective remains controversial. One of the controversies has been centered around the choice of type of exercise, varying between flexion, extension, aerobic, stretching for flexibility, and strengthening.

The emphasis on the benefit of exercise has the following intentions: (a) strengthen and increase endurance of the spinal muscles, (b) reduce mechanical stress by improving ergonomics, (c) correct posture, and (d) ultimately reduce or eliminate pain.

Increasing strength and endurance of the back and abdominal muscles became the cornerstone of exercise for the low back, providing that the appropriate muscles are exercised. General conditioning exercises then can be done for whatever purpose those exercises demand.

Specific Exercise Protocols

Walking as an exercise prescription is probably the simplest, least stressful, and most beneficial therapeutic exercise for the low back. In proper walking there is contralateral swing of the arms, which causes a physiologic rotation of the trunk at each step. As physiologic rotation of each functional unit occurs, the collagen fibers of that layer and therefore of that angulation are extended, which strengthens them.

Flexibility

Although "range of motion" is difficult to document objectively, flexibility of the spinal segment needs attention. Flexibility occurs in the soft tissues of the spine: the muscles and their fascia, the tendons, ligaments, and facet joint capsules. All these tissues are composed of collagen fibers, fibrous and elastin tissues that have a physiologic elongation that must be maintained by repeated active and passive stretching. The annular fibers of the discs also consist of type I collagen fibers with some type II and need physiologic elongation. Flexibility thus aims also at improving disc nutrition.

The response of tissue to elongation activities can be summarized as follows (53):

1. Collagen fibers that are elongated 1% to 1.5% for less than 1 hour show no permanent deformation (elongation).
2. Elongation of 1.5% to 2% maintained for more than 1 hour will result in permanent elongation, as that degree of stretch results in a melting of the tropocollagen bonds. This gain is lost if elongation is less than 1 hour or if the tissues are allowed to lose their elongation.
3. Elongation of 2% may allow a return to prestretch length if not followed by sustained or intermittent stretch during the subsequent 24 hours.
4. Elongation of 3% to 8% may cause a loss of continuity of the collagen fibers and result in structural damage.

5. Permanent stretching or excessive elongation of the collagen fibers disrupts the intermolecular bonds between the tropocollagen units, causing permanent damage.

Heating the tissues facilitates flexibility. Any treatment program to increase flexibility is indicated. The application of heat must be gentle and progressive. Rapid stretching must be controlled as well as the extent of stretch. The lack of daily flexibility activities causes a significant loss of dense connective-tissue strength and elasticity. After any injury to the soft tissues of the spine, elongation exercises must be initiated, keeping in mind the biomechanical properties of collagen fibers. This indicates slow, prolonged stretching exercises of the specific muscle (fascia) found to be limited on clinical examination. Active exercises are safer and more effective than are passive exercises. Flexibility exercises must include rotational as well as sagittal motion.

The lumbar zygapophyseal joints limit axial rotation to about 1 degree at each lumbar level on each side, so repeated rotations exceeding 1 degree could cause microdamage to the facets and the intervertebral discs, but this has not been confirmed in normal discs.

Strengthening Exercises

Exercises of all muscles involved in normal trunk activity, whether those involving stability or kinetic action, must be instituted to restore and maintain strength and endurance. The abdominal flexor muscle have been clearly designated as those mostly needing strengthening. Of the abdominal flexors muscles, the deep abdominal muscles and the quadratus lumbar muscles unload the spine and thus deserve emphasis.

The exercises recommended to strengthen the deep abdominal muscles, especially the transversus muscles, are shown in (Figs. 7.8 through 7.11). "Tilting the pelvis" (decreasing the lumbar lordosis) is indicated as an exercise, this must be performed in the standing position and must be incorporated in any lifting activity, as the tilting stabilizes the low back.

The other muscles that stabilize the low back are those of the quadratus lumborum. These are strengthened by lying on one's side and upon the dependent elbow. The entire body is then elevated laterally and held there for increasing periods of time (Fig. 7.12). In patients with clinical evidence of discogenic disease with pain radiating down the leg, indicating possible disc herniation, lumbar flexion would appear to be contraindicated, as this movement apparently herniates the disc nucleus further posteriorly against the posterior longitudinal ligament and the nerve roots in the foramen. The stabilizing exercises described earlier and done properly are not flexion exercises but stabilizing exercises.

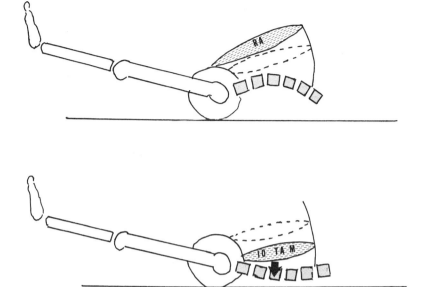

FIG. 7.8. Exercise to strengthen the transversus muscles. With two-leg elevation to approximately 4 to 6 inches the rectus abdominis muscles (RA) contract, but when the deep muscles are weak (*dotted lines*), the back arches and the stability of the spine do not increase. Bottom figure shows that with the elevation of the legs and intentional "flattening" of the low back against the floor, the internal oblique (IO) and the transversus abdominal muscles (TAM) contract. These stabilize the trunk.

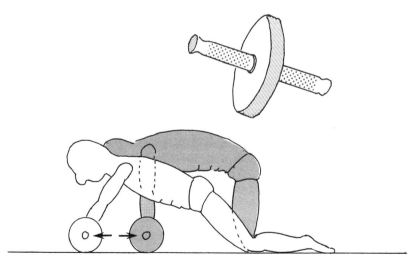

FIG. 7.9. "Roller" exercises for deep abdominal muscles. Using a single wheel roller starting from the fully flexed position (shaded figure), the roller is pushed further and returned. As the wheel goes further the abdominal muscles contract with increased strength.

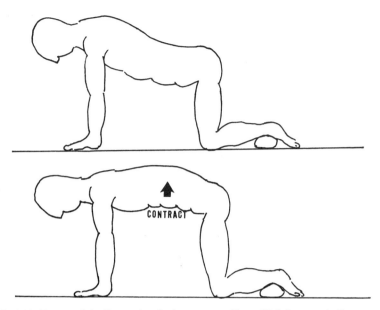

FIG. 7.10. Prone pelvic tilt exercise. In the prone position with balance on both arms and legs the low back "sags," then elevates, and is held there for increasing periods of time.

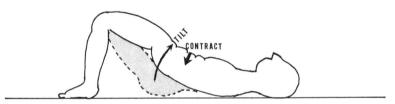

FIG. 7.11. Supine pelvic tilting exercise. In the supine position with both legs flexed the pelvis is elevated while keeping the low back against the floor. This is not elevating the entire low back, which would arch the lumbar spine. Proper pelvic tilting activates the deep abdominal flexor muscles. Repeated tilting increases endurance as well as strength.

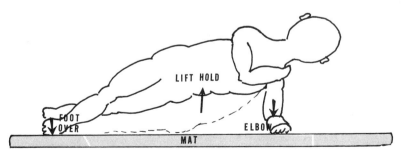

FIG. 7.12. Quadratus lumborum exercise. On the side-lying position and up on the dependent elbow, the entire body is slowly elevated and held there for increasing periods of time.

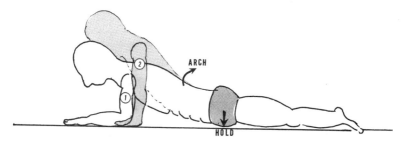

FIG. 7.13. Mackenzie extension exercise. In the prone position the patient elevates the upper body, passively extending the low back. Elevation to support the body on the elbows is followed by elevating the body to full arm extension. The effort is active with the arms and passive with the low back extensors.

MacKenzie (54) agreed and postulated that lumbosacral extension caused the nucleus to migrate anteriorly and away from sensitive neural tissues capable of causing low back pain and sciatica. He thus postulated extension exercises to accomplish this mechanism (Fig. 7.13). MRI studies have confirmed migration of the nucleus. The current approach is to use the extension test of MacKenzie to determine the change of symptoms. When low back pain and sciatica diminish from the extension exercise, gentle, gradual flexion exercises and other exercises to increase flexibility, strength, and proper body mechanics should be included. This treatment protocol is widespread today and awaits assessment of outcome.

Back School

The "Back School" which was intended to instruct the person in how to properly bend, lift, stoop, push, pull, and so on, has failed to change the incidence of low back injuries in industry. Farfan (55) stated, "It is very interesting how many interested men . . . do not agree that back pain is preventable or even controllable with back school methods. Many back schools . . . are simply exercise programs and audiovisual programs." He then went on to state, "back schools are for education and training using the principle of body mechanics and back health care for prevention and control of back pain in the most efficient manner."

These statements indicate that many so-called back schools do not embody the concept of a school. All exercises are useless if the principles of proper body mechanics are not done daily. Most deviations from normal involve the presence of perturbers, which upset the proper body mechanics that are discovered during back school sessions (56–59).

Ergonomics (60) has held a prominent place in proper body mechanics. Ergonomics is defined as, "The science concerned with how to fit a job to man's anatomical, physiologic and psychologic characteristics in a way that will enhance human efficiency and well-being." Recently, Congress has studied grants for further OSHA research because, "The scientific evidence supporting the new ergonomic standard is sketchy and flawed. It is inconclusive and extremely complex" (61). The ergonomics regarding low back care is equally complex and inconclusive. Activities must be tailored to the specific needs of a person with a specific job requirement; often this is not fully understood or evaluated. Perturbers, such as fatigue, anger, anxiety, impatience, depression, and boredom, may interfere with normal neuromuscular efficiency and may vary from day today, which makes it difficult to incorporate into a back school.

Most ergonomic assessments in the workplace have focused on the postures of the worker and the loads imposed upon a joint because of these postures but have ignored the influence of dynamic motion on joint loading. These dynamic forces relate to velocity, acceleration, and muscular coactivation of the trunk musculature (62). These factors may not have been employed but a recent large-scale, randomized, controlled trial of educational programs to prevent work-associated low back injuries found no long-term benefit from the training (60).

In evaluating ergonomic conditions it must always be remembered that prolonged or repetitive flexed position has been shown to cause "creep" in the soft tissues of function units: ligaments, disc annular fibers, and capsules of facets. This creep increases the laxity and thus impairs stability, with consequent injury and associated pain.

This increased laxity is not essentially in the ligaments or in the capsules of the facets but is considered to be due to a decrease in the height of the disc as a result of dehydration. The fluid content of the disc changes over a 24-hour period, which is aggravated by prolonged flexion both in standing and in sitting. These prolonged and repetitive (cyclic) flexed positions are used frequently in individuals who sustain industrial injuries.

The muscles that maintain stability become fatigued from the flexed cyclic and/or sustained posture from impairment of the spinal ligamento-muscular reflex due to fatigue of the mechanoreceptors in the ligaments (62).

Because lifting in industry has caused low back disorders, safe lifting methods have been offered, but they have not yet led to improved results. Squat lifting (Fig. 7.14) has been considered the safest way to lift, but the best posture of the lumbar spine during the lift remains unclear. A kyphotic posture of the lumbosacral spine has been recommended because it allegedly places the stress upon the posterior ligaments that have great resiliency, whereas in the lordotic posture (Fig. 7.15) these ligaments are relaxed.

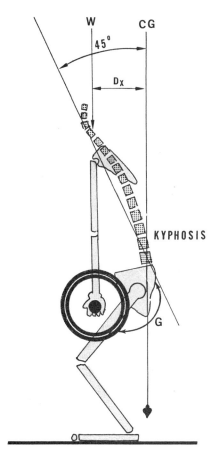

FIG. 7.14. Squat-lifting technique with kyphotic lumbar spine. The standard squat lift is shown with the weight (W) being lifted some distance (Dx) from the center of gravity (CG). This is postulated to impose the stress upon the ligamentous tissues.

Intermittent Rest Periods

The first 10 minutes of rest after cyclic loading provide some recovery, but full recovery is impossible after twice as long a period as that of the cyclic or prolonged period. Periodic periods of rest of sufficient duration must be instituted in industrial settings that require prolonged or cyclic flexed position. This is not frequently encouraged or mandated (60).

PSYCHOLOGIC ASPECTS OF LOW BACK DISORDERS

In a recent series of articles (61,62) the authors "took aim at several common misconceptions about back pain and back disabilities." They contest the notion that back pain among workers typically results from an injury. "There is very little evidence that most back pain stems from a discrete injury or repetitive trauma" (62). They further state, "the experience profoundly depends on whether the individual has the ability to cope with the episode."

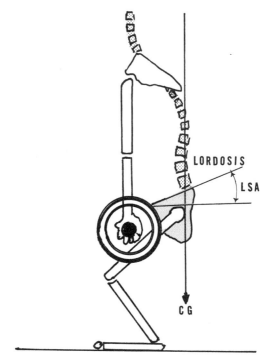

FIG. 7.15. Squat lift with maintained lordosis. The squat lift shown maintains lumbar lordosis by increasing the lumbosacral angle (LSA).

This concept adds credence to the statement made earlier in this text that the emotional status of the person "before" the painful disabling incidence—whether anxiety, impatience, fatigue or even depression—strongly influences the performance of the neuromuscular activity. The preceding finding by Hadler et al. further implicates the interpretation of the significance of the pain. The relationship of the patient with the physician is paramount in the possibility of chronic pain. As stated by Hadler, "The social construction of ascribing disabling regional back pain to an injury is potentially iatrogenic and likely to have lasting effects on the individual's sense of invincibility."

There is little evidence that altering physical demands of work or the physical condition of the person has a major impact on the prevalence of back pain or back disability (61). Proper management of the patient with acute low back symptoms must keep these acts in mine. Pain, its mechanism, and its significance must be explained to the patient as well as treated.

Pain occurring from the low back has been depicted as the low back disorder being a "neuro-muscular-skeletal-psychologic entity," which implies that the psychologic aspect is causative and/or a result of ineffectively treated low back disorders. The patient's reaction to this persistent disorder leads to chronic pain that persists after the objective aspects of the condition have disappeared.

Treatment of chronic pain is not the main objective of this text. However, as low back pain resulting from mechanical disorder is currently accepted, some discussion of pain perception is warranted. Disability resulting from pain must be viewed from a cognitive–behavioral perspective influenced by organic pathology and motoric-environmental factors (62–66). Numerous studies have shown a relationship between psychosocial and behavioral factors and pain, impairment, and resultant disability (67–70). This unfortunately has led many uninformed examiners to assume that the resultant pain is psychologic, without a mechanical or organic basis, when both are pertinent.

In the neurologic sequence schemata proposed in Fig. 1.0 any psychologic factor, such as anger, impatience, anxiety, or depression, can alter the sequence and act as a perturber. In this context a psychologic factor can alter the mechanical function and lead to a low back disorder. This does not imply that any resultant pain is psychologic, but it suggests that psychologic factors can impair normal function and result in pain. When a perturber persists or is excessive, acute pain becomes chronic, although there is no evidence of further tissue damage (70–73).

When a person is confronted with a stressor there is an instant automatic sympathetic arousal which diminishes that person's ability to tolerate the pain, resulting in reduced function (74). This sympathetic arousal displays an elevation of electromyographic activity of the paraspinous muscles, which contributes to the impaired function (75).

A cognitive–perceptual response to a stressor is the way a person perceives and interprets the effect upon his or her relationship to the environment and control over that change. When pain becomes a sign of a serious health problem, it is considered an illness (76). The interpretation now has greater, and different, significance.

The avoidance of activity, fear of movement, or fear of work-related activities may persist as a result of the acute pain. This excessive and often irrational fear of physical movement has been termed *kinesophobia* (77–79).

In evaluating cognition of the resultant pain from a low back disorder that becomes chronic, the question of what patients think of their pain is thus pertinent. A questionnaire of 50 questions (Pain Cognitive List) has been proposed (77) and should be considered when a patient exhibits chronicity in symptoms in spite of appropriate treatment.

Cognitive behavioral therapy remains unfamiliar to many physicians and therapists. This therapeutic approach begins immediately upon physician–therapist–patient encounter (80,81). The interpretation of subjective symptoms, objective examination, and interpretation (for the patient) of laboratory findings contribute to the patient's understanding of the illness. Physicians are mostly trained in the biomedical model and are less comfortable with the psychosocial aspects of illness (82–86). As Vlaeyen and Linton state, "For many patients the physician represents a formidable source of power and influence" (87).

The cognitive–behavioral principle aims to mediate change in attitudes and behaviors upon recognizing (cognition) all aspects of low back disorders in meaningful terms. The term *nonorganic* postulated by Waddell (85) has become an accepted test to implicate psychologic variants in illness behavior, but it should also implement cognitive principles, as excessive emotional behavior is often based on improper or inadequate cognition.

Many patients with low back disorders unfortunately become the "undesirable patient" (86), defined by the following traits:

1. Socially undesirable, including alcoholics, uneducated, dirty, aged, or very poor.
2. Undesirable attitudes, such as ungrateful attitude, defiance, or failure to accept the knowledge or impression of the physician. The patient who "wants to know too much" or "thinks he knows too much."
3. Apparent absence of a physical illness or the presence of many illnesses that complicate the primary complaint.
4. Circumstantial undesirability, such as being tardy for an appointment or unaccepting of the manner of payment.

These "undesirable" patients unfortunately are so labeled and therefore do not get appropriate care.

Evaluation of the patient who exhibits kinesiophobia has been proposed by the Dutch Version Testing (84). When asked these questions their answer indicates what compliance the physician can expect from any therapeutic attempt and indicates what assurance or expectation the patient be given.

1. I am afraid that I may injure myself if I exercise.
2. If I were to try to overcome (my impairment), my pain would increase.
3. My body is telling me that I have something dangerously wrong.
4. My pain would probably be relieved if I were to exercise.
5. People are not taking my medical condition seriously.
6. My accident has put my body at risk for the rest of my life.
7. Pain always means I have injured my body.
8. Just because something aggravates my pain does not mean it i dangerous.

9. I am afraid that I might injure myself accidentally.
10. Simply being careful that I do not make unnecessary movements is the safest thing I can do to prevent my pain from worsening.
11. I would not have this much pain if there were not something potentially dangerous going on in my body.
12. Although my condition is painful I would be better off if I were physically active.
13. Pain lets me know when to stop exercising so that I do not injure myself.
14. It is really not safe for a person with a condition like mine to be physically active.
15. I cannot do all the things normal people do because it is too easy for me to get injured.
16. Even though something is causing me a lot of pain I do not think it is actually dangerous.
17. No one should have to exercise when he/she is in pain.

The reaction to these simple statements gives the examiner an idea of the patient's understanding of his or her low back problem and justifies implementing a cognitive approach. This is particularly true as "fear avoidance," the fear of pain and its possible recurrence, has been viewed as a basis for disability rather than acute pain, and for acute pain becoming chronic after the acute injury has healed (87–91). A recent article in the *Annals of Internal Medicine* advocated stepped care for back pain, involving the primary care physician in encouraging patients to resume their normal daily activities (92).

In their three stages the major approach was to assure the patient that low back pain is not necessarily debilitating and that resuming normal activities is not detrimental or impairing and therefore should not be avoided. All three phases discuss the avoidance of fear and advise treatment of the "psychological illness presented by the symptom of fear from the low back."

This has been paramount in the standard care of the patient with low back pain. Taking x-rays, which usually are uninformative, implies the possibility of a structural and therefore an "untreatable condition." Such terms as "degenerative disc disease" indicate to the patient that the condition is "degenerative" and involves a disease, none of which is pertinent.

The advice to rest and avoid certain positions and activities is usually also not founded on any scientific basis and is erroneously interpreted by the patient as ominous. Any medication should be explained as being directed at the symptom, and not at the condition. Any prognosis given the patient should be the natural history of most low back complaints. The patient should be assured that any program is merely to hasten recovery and prevent recurrence, which is the major fear.

Chronic pain remains as confused as it is misunderstood. Impairment from chronic pain involves local tissue damage, injury to the central nervous system, affect state, and interaction with the environment (93).

CONCLUSION

Lumbar pain and radiculopathy have a favorable prognosis in most patients. Active care is more effective than passive care. Relief of pain in the acute phase is mandatory to permit the patient to become actively involved. A full understanding by the patient and reassurance by the physician ensure compliance. Avoidance of frightening words depicting the diagnosis, which is partially unknown by the physician and threatening to the patient, almost ensures chronicity as a result of failure of appropriate early care by the physician. Inappropriate use and explanation of radiologic studies often confuse the patient and misinform the treating physician. Prolonged bed rest should be avoided, as it induces muscular atrophy and psychological deterioration.

Within 3 months or less a natural recovery of an acute low back disorder occurs regardless of the treatment. Thus surgery is rarely indicated before 6 to 12 weeks, and then depends on the progression of objective neurologic changes. Surgery rarely eliminates pain unless there is a tissue change that causes the pain and can be remedied by surgical intervention. The use of many modalities, such as manipulation, mobilization, traction, acupuncture, and other modalities, can be helpful, provided it is done within a reasonable time, for good reason, and with objective results. Many of these alternative forms of treatment can cause dependency and prolongation of impairment. Mere failure of subjective improvement by these conservative approaches is not an indication for surgical intervention.

Even though randomized controlled studies have refuted the benefit of an educational program known as Back School, they in no way diminish the benefit of teaching the patient what the problem is in meaningful words and offering participation in an active program that places the patient in charge.

Low back pain is the commonest cause of limited activities among people under the age of 45 and one of the commonest reasons for seeking health care. The cause of low back pain is unknown but is generally thought to be multifactorial—including physical, legal, socioeconomic, and psychologic—and hence to be an "enigma." It cannot be viewed as only a medical problem; instead it should be viewed as a biologic–psychologic–social complex.

Surgical intervention in the treatment of low back pain with or without radiculitis has not been discussed, but the benefit of surgical intervention remains questionable in some aspects but valid in others.

As an example of the enigmas involving surgical intervention, the concept that instability is a major cause of low back impairment and thus that stabilizing the site of instability (fusion) is beneficial appears substantiated (90).

Radiographic evidence of instability often does not correlate with the patient's symptoms or comply with the traditional biomechanical definition of instability. The healthy spine allows motion at all levels. Fusion is not physiologic (89), as it carries the risk of disruption to the functioning of the entire spinal column, especially the function of adjacent units above or below. Other modalities that are considered to be standard treatment demand further unbiased and controlled studies. The enigma of the low back remains controversial and not fully accepted by all professionals whose main concern is the care of the impaired patient.

More recently, medical treatment is assuming a greater role as the standard forms of treatment have failed to afford the results expected. Conservative treatment protocols, as listed earlier, help most patients weather their symptoms while sciatica runs its course. Patients with protracted sciatica, however, fail to receive the needed or expected relief from conservative treatments, and this is true even of surgical intervention.

Surgical intervention is not the ideal treatment for disc herniations that incite mechanical compression of the nerve but fail to relieve the chemical aspects of nerve roots inflammation. Researchers in Sweden (93) have shown that chemical intervention using a monoclonal antibody (termed *infliximab*) relieved pain from the inflamed nerve root. This inflammation is known to result from a chemical cause, identified as tumor necrosis factor alpha (TNF-alpha). This chemical relief, blocking the activity of TNF-alpha, prevents damage to the nerve.

So far these findings have been observed in animal experiments only, with a limited application in humans, and this treatment is very expensive. However, this appears to be a long-needed breakthrough in meaningful care of painful protracted sciatica. There are also side effects that will need to be corrected or modified, but this approach to the care of sciatica from herniated lumbar discs remains promising. The timing of the use of TNF-alpha remains unresolved, as in animal studies the drug was administered at the time of injury, which would be difficult in humans.

Also, TNF-alpha may interfere with the body's normal process of resorption. Many more studies must be conducted in humans, but these preliminary studies indicate potential benefit from chemical treatment. This possibility does not refute all the modalities and indications referred to earlier.

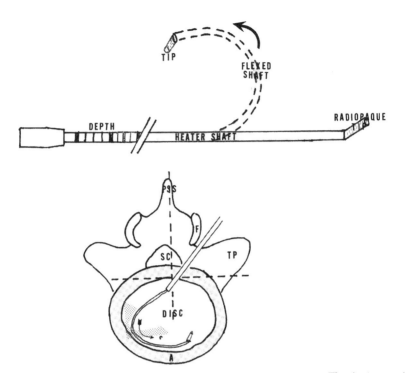

FIG. 7.16. Iintradiscal electrothermal therapy instrumentation. The instrument shows the rigid shaft and its depth determination with the flexible heater shaft and its radio-opaque tip, which shows where the shaft is during the procedure shown below. The lower part of the figure shows how the instrument is inserted between the foramen (F) and the transverse process (TP) until it reaches the annulus (A) and curves around the disc. PSS, posterior superior spine; SC, the spinal canal.

In place of surgical intervention, intradiscal electrothermal therapy (IDET) was proposed, and initially considered a valid treatment when all else failed. This procedure cannot be considered noninvasive because it involves inserting a navigable catheter into the disc. The catheter proceeds circumferentially around the disc and then is heated by an external monitor to a temperature that alters the collagen fibers, stiffens the disc, and ablates the nociceptors (Figs. 7.16 and 7.17). With the "dehydration" and essential "denervation" of the disc, almost instant relief of pain and impairment was originally claimed.

Conflicting results are now reported, which makes the procedure still indicated, but with better controls (94–98). A recent article in *Spine* (99) indicates that 2 years after being treated with IDET, patients demonstrated statistically significant improvement in pain, clinical function, and quality of life.

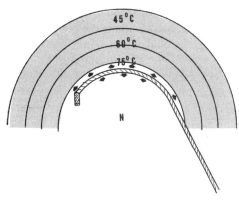

FIG. 7.17. Heat generated in gradients. With controlled heat the inner annulus receives 75°C with the more outer layers receiving increasing lysis the nucleus.

The mechanical aspect of spinal radiculopathy was initially considered the principal cause, until chemical expression from the damaged spinal tissues was seen as contributing to the resultant pain from the mechanical pressure. Animal models and experimentation are casting some light on mechanisms previously suspected but not clearly defined. Using the Kawakami-Weinstein rat model of radiculopathy, the following questions arose:

1. What is the effect of isolating the root injury to a single L5 spinal level?
2. Can a focal mechanical injury without exogenous inflammatory mediator induce pain in the rat?
3. Can a vertebral disc herniation with mechanical compression of a root be effective without direct application of autologous or nonautologous disc material?
4. What are the similarities between central (root) and peripheral (nerve) injuries on spinal glial activation and proinflammatory cytokine expression?
5. What is the impact of root injury on the spinal cord?

The answers to questions 1 to 3 are obviously negative from current thinking, but Deleo et al. (96), having concentrated on questions 4 and 5 with promising deduction, are discovering a new mechanism for pain (100). Inflammation, which is the basis for pain, acute and chronic, is a physiologic process by which all vascularized tissues respond to injury. During this process, soluble and cellular mediators collaborate to contain and/or eliminate the agents causing the physical symptoms. In proper proportion, this process is beneficial for survival of the tissue, but when uncontrolled, they can cause serious damage.

Inflammation is divided into acute and chronic response, with the acute phase being rapid, being short-lived, and consisting of edema, invasion of plasma proteins and neutrophil leukocytes. Chronic inflammation, on the other hand, lasts longer and involves the invasion of lymphocyte macrophages and fibroblasts.

The soluble proinflammatory mediators increase blood flow, vascular permeability, migration of leukocytes into the injured tissues, and activation of these leukocytes to eliminate the invading substances. Among these soluble mediators are protease systems, peptides, lipids, and especially cytokines. (The latter are DeLeo's concern.)

The acute inflammatory molecular mediators are well documented and include plasma protease, complement, kinins, clotting fibronolytic proteins, lipids, prostaglandins, leukotrienes, peptides, neuropeptides, nitric oxide, and cytokines. These cytokines are now implemented in persistent chronic pain.

The cytokine interleukin-6 (Il-6) is presently being thoroughly investigated, although all the preceding are involved to a degree in chronic pain. Il-6 is produced by the T-lymphocytes, endothelial cells, monocytes, and fibroblasts promoting monocytic differentiation, increasing the number of platelets and synthesis of fibrinogen.

When acute inflammation persists, chronic inflammation takes over. The neutrophils are replaced by macrophages, lymphocytes, and fibroblasts. Cytokines are also expressed. Their role in influencing the nervous system is currently under scrutiny (101). Local release of cytokines directs the process of peripheral nerve degeneration and regeneration.

Neuropathic pain, especially chronic pain, has remained refractory to the usual medication and techniques, which has promoted the study of the influence of cytokines. Il-6 is produced distal to the injury site of a peripheral nerve, but its origin in the spinal cord remains unknown, although CNS microglia and astrocytes produce Il-6 in response to injury (102–106).

Cytokines are produced in the periphery by microphages and Schwann cells (Figs. 7.18 and 7.19). Axonal flow is well recognized (Fig. 7.20). After injury to a peripheral nerve there is retrograde flow via axonal or nonaxonal routes into the dorsal root ganglion and to the dorsal horn of the cord. Specific cytokines may also be produced within hours in the spinal cord by the activated microglia, astrocytes, and other pathway neurons. All these factors have a serious impact on understanding the mechanism of pain transmission and the onset of chronicity and persistence (Fig. 7.21).

Pressure, loose ligature, and ice send cytokines retrograde to the cord, where glial cells in the cord (Fig. 7.22), both dorsal horn (sensory) and anterior horn cells (motor), express cytokines. These cytokines are

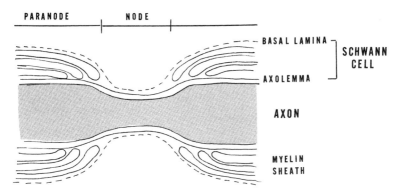

FIG. 7.18. Schwann cell. The Schwann cell is shown with its components and the node.

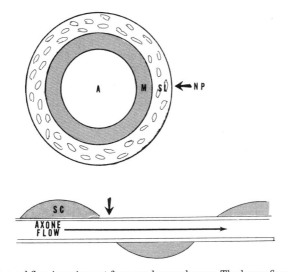

FIG. 7.19. Axonal flow impairment from nucleus pulposus. The lower figure shows the axonal flow within a Schwann cell (SC). The upper figure shows how the nucleus pulposus (NP) chemically encroaches upon the Schmidt-Lanterman (SL) incisure, causing swelling that compresses the myelin (M) and in turn compresses the axon (A) and decreases flow.

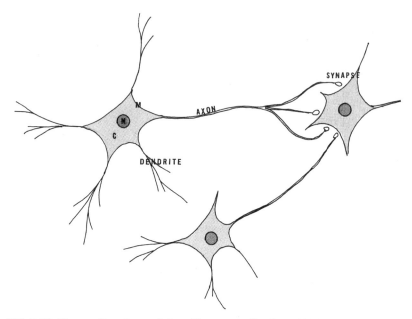

FIG. 7.20. Nerve cell and axonal flow. The nerve cell is bounded by a membrane (M) that contains the cytoplasm (C) and its nucleus (N). Each cell has an axon and multiple dendrites that connect (synapse) with numerous other cells.

considered to originate from monocytes that have invaded the area via inflammation (106–108).

BIOLOGIC TREATMENT OF SCIATICA

Treatment of sciatic radiculopathy that is consistent with the recent discovery of chemokines has recently been postulated. Swedish researchers have reported a biologic treatment for sciatica (109) that remains to be confirmed by further studies but promises new understanding of inflammation for discal damage.

With one infusion of infliximab, a powerful antiinflammatory agent, these researchers eliminated the symptoms of sciatica. This agent, a monoclonal antibody, blocks the activity of TNF-alpha, a cytokine that appears to play a significant role in inflammation of the sciatic nerve. Further studies are necessary (110,111) before its daily use can be advocated, but this does not refute the emergence of cytokines as being involved in sciatic neuropathy.

To supplement the preceding article, another has appeared demonstrating that inflammatory infiltrates (monocytes and macrophages) into herniated lumbar discs exist in an inactive state. These infiltrates are recruited (regulated) through interaction with specific chemo-

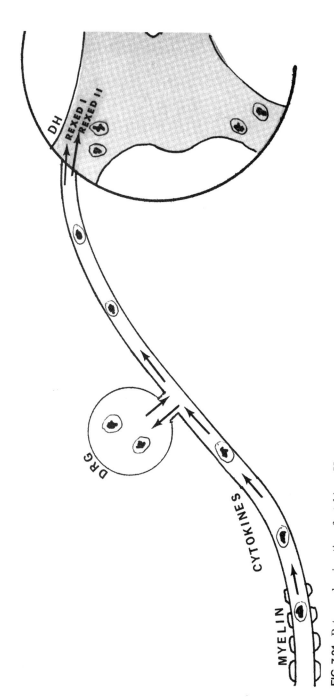

FIG. 7.21. Retrograde migration of cytokines. Upon trauma to the peripheral nerve the myelin "secretes" cytokines that retrograde migrate to the dorsal horn cell (DH) of the cord and stimulate the Rexed layers I and II (substantia gelatinosum).

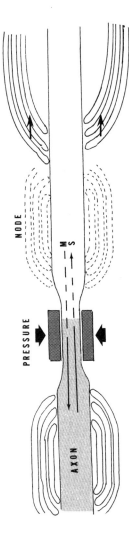

FIG. 7.22. Axonal pressure. Pressure behind or between nodes expresses cytokines affecting sensory (S) and motor (M) nerves. (From Figure 1.9 in Cailliet R. Soft tissue pain and disability. Philadelphia: FA Davis, 1996. with permission.)

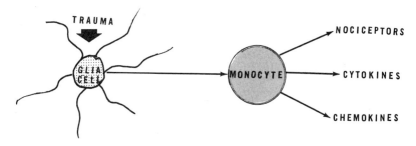

FIG. 7.23. Trauma stimulating cytokines. Trauma to the glial cells of discs initiates secretion of kines from monocytes.

attractants (chemokines and extracellular matrix proteins). Of these chemokines 44 are known and classified into CXC, CC, C, and CX3C subfamilies that exert their chemoattraction via G protein–coupled receptors on the cell surfaces. One of these chemokines is 1 MCP-1/CCI2, which is found in intervertebral discs (112,114). In resorption of herniated disc material the mechanism postulated macrophages as playing a leading role. How these macrophages accumulate into the disc remains unclear. Human intervertebral discs have intrinsic chemoattractants—chemokines—that attract monocytes. Herniation of a disc (Fig. 7.23), especially if associated with microinvasion of vessels, recruits circulating monocytes from the bloodstream into the disc. These monocytes may secrete chemokines that affect the structure of the disc. More knowledge will emerge, but it is now clear that there is a specific chemical pathogenesis to disc disease and that in the future the mechanical aspects of treatment will be replaced by antichemical intervention involving cytokines.

REFERENCES

1. Loeser JD. The future: will pain be abolished or just pain management specialists? *Pain: Clinical Updates* 2000;8:1–4.
2. Bonica JJ. *The management of pain.* Philadelphia: Lea & Febiger, 1953.
3. Thomas CL, ed. *Taber's cyclopedic medical dictionary,* 16th ed. Philadelphia: FA Davis, 1989.
4. *Guides to the evaluation of permanent impairment,* 4th ed. Chicago: American Medical Association, 1993.
5. Merskey H, Bogduk N, eds. *Classification of chronic pain: description of chronic pain syndromes and definition of pain terms.* Report by the International Association for the Study of Pain Task Force on Taxonomy, 2nd ed. Seattle: IASP Press, 1994.
6. Anand KJS, Rovnaghi C, Walden M, et al. Consciousness behavior and clinical impact on the definition of pain. *Pain Forum* 1999;8:64–73.
7. Rollman GB. Competent treatment in the absence of a universal definition of pain. *Pain Forum* 1999;8:103–105.

8. Van Tulder MW, Koes BW, Bouter LM. Conservative treatment of acute and chronic nonspecific low back pain. *Spine* 1997;22:2128–2156.
9. Federation of State Medical Boards of the United States. *Model guidelines for the use of controlled substances for the treatment of pain.* Euless, TX: The Federation, 1998.
10. Carr DB, Goudas LC. Acute pain, *Lancet* 1999;353:2051–2058.
11. Atkinson JH, Slater MA, Epping-Jordan JE. Identifying individuals at risk for chronicity. *Pain Forum* 1997;6:137–139.
12. Jamison RN, Rudy TE, Penzien DB, et al. Cognitive-behavioral classifications of chronic pain: replication and extension of empirically defined patient profiles. *Pain* 1994;57:249–283.
13. Klapow JC, Slater MA, Patterson TL, et al. An empirical evaluation of multidimensional clinic outcome in chronic low back pain patients. *Pain* 1993;55:107–118.
14. Klapow JC, Slater MA, Patterson TL, et al. Psychosocial factors discriminate multidimensional clinic groups of chronic low back pain patients. *Pain* 1995;62:349–355.
15. Turk DC, Rudy TE. The robustness of an empirically derived taxonomy of chronic pain patients. *Pain* 1990;43:27–35.
16. Von Korff M, Dworkin SF, LeResche L. Graded chronic pain status: an epidemiologic evaluation. *Pain* 1990;40:279–291.
17. Flores L, Gatchek RJ, Polatin PB. Objectification of functional improvement after nonoperative care. *Spine* 1997;22:1622–1633.
18. Woolf CJ, Mannion R. Neuropathic pain: aetiology, symptoms, mechanisms, and management. *Lancet* 1999;353:1959–1964.
19. Benson JM. The neurobiology of pain. *Lancet* 1999;353:1610–1615.
20. Devor M. Unexplained peculiarities of the dorsal root ganglion, *Pain* 1999(Suppl 6);S27–S35.
21. Melzack R, Wall PD. Pain mechanisms: a new theory. *Science* 1965;150:971–979.
22. Levine J, Taiwo Y. Inflammatory pain. In: Wall PD, Melzack R, eds. *Textbook of pain.* Edinburgh: Churchill Livingstone, 1994:45–56.
23. Loeser JD, Melzack R. Pain: an overview *Lancet* 1999;353:1607–1609.
24. Dubner R, Ruda MA. Activity-dependent neuronal plasticity following tissue injury and inflammation. *Trends Neurosci* 1992:15:96–103.
25. Gracely RH, Lynch SA, Bennett GH. Painful neuropathy: altered central processing maintained by peripheral input. *Pain* 1992:51:175–194.
26. Rainville P, Duncan GH, Price DD, et al. Selective modulation of pain unpleasantness alters activity in the human cerebral cortex. *Neurosci Abstr* 1996:614:2.
27. Melzack R. Phantom limbs and the concept of a neuromatrix. *Trends Neurosci* 1990:13:88–92.
28. LeDoux JE. Emotions, memory and the brain. *Sci Am* 1994;270:50–57.
29. LeDoux JE. Sensory systems and emotions: a model of affective processing. *Integr Psychiatry* 1986:4:237–248.
30. McCormack K. Non-steroidal anti-inflammatory drugs and spinal nociceptive processing. *Pain* 1994;59:9–44.
31. McQuay H. Opioids in pain management. *Lancet* 1999;353:2229–2232.
32. Dilke TF, Burry HC, Grahame R. Epidural corticosteroid in injection in management of lumbar root compression. *Br Med J* 1973:162:653–657.
33. Clayton L. Thomas, ed. *Taber's cyclopedic medical dictionary,* 16th ed. Philadelphia: FA Davis, 1989:1409.

34. Gammon GD, Starr I. Studies on the relief of pain by counter-irritation. *J Physiol* 1993;72:392.
35. Douglas WW, Malcolm JL. The effect of localized cooling on conduction in cat nerves. *J Physiol* 1955;130:53.
36. Li-L. Effect of cooling on neuromuscular transmission in the rat. *Am J Physiol* 194:200, 1958.
37. Lehmann JF, DeLateur BJ. Therapeutic heat. In: Lehmann JF, ed. *Therapeutic heat and cold,* 4th ed. Baltimore: Williams & Wilkins, 1989.
38. Michlovitz SL. Biophysical principles of heating and superficial heat agents. In: Michlovitz SL, ed. *Thermal agents in rehabilitation.* Philadelphia: FA Davis, 1990.
39. Currier DP, Kramer JF. Sensory nerve conduction: heating effects of ultrasound and infrared. *Physiother Can* 1982;34:241.
40. Hadler NM, Curtis P, Gillings DB, et al. A benefit of spinal manipulation an adjunctive therapy for acute low back pain: a stratified controlled trial. *Spine* 1987:12:702–706.
41. Shekelle PG, Aams AH, Chassin MR, et al. Spinal manipulation for low back pain. *Br Med J* 1992:117:590–598.
42. Larsson U, Choler U, Lidstrom A et al. Auto-traction for treatment of lumbago-sciatica. *Acta Othop Scand* 1980;51:791–843.
43. Mathews JA, Hickling J. Lumbar traction: a double-blind controlled study for sciatica. *Rheumatol Rehab* 1975:14:222–225.
44. Onel D, Tuzlaci M, Sari H, et al. Computed tomographic investigation of the effect of traction on lumbar disc herniations. *Spine* 1989:14:82–90.
45. Robison R. The new back school prescription: stabilization training. Part 1: *Occup Med* 1992;7:17–31.
46. Saal JA, Saal JS. Non-operative treatment of herniated disc with radiculopathy: an outcome study. *Spine* 1989;14:431–437.
47. Bergmark A. Stability of the lumbar spine: a study in mechanical engineering. *Acta Orthop Scand* (Suppl) 1989;230:20–24.
48. Cholewichi J, Panjabi MM, Khachatryan L. Stabilizing function of trunk flexor-extensor muscles around a neutral spine posture. *Spine* 1997;22:2207–2212.
49. White AA, Panjabi MM. Clinical biomechanics of the spine, 2nd Edition. Philadelphia: J.B. Lippincott, 1990:278–378.
50. Jayson MIV. Why does acute back pain become chronic? *Spine* 1997;22: 1053–1056.
51. Saal JS. The role of inflammation. *Spine* 1995:20:1821–1827.
52. Kimori H, Shimimiya K, Nakai O, et al. The natural history of herniated nucleus pulposus with radiculopathy. *Spine* 1996:21:225–229.
53. Tillman LJ, Cummings GS. Biological mechanisms of connective tissue mutability. In: Currier DP, Nelson RM. *Dynamics of human biologic tissues.* Philadelphia: FA Davis, 1992:1–44.
54. MacKenzie RA. *The lumbar spine: mechanical diagnosis and therapy.* Waikanae, New Zealand: Spinal Publications, 1981.
55. Farfan WH. Personal communication, July 4, 1979.
56. Daltroy LH, Iverson MR, Larson MG, et al. A controlled trial of an educational program to prevent low back injuries. *N Engl J Med* 1997;337: 322–328
57. Bitter debate over ergonomics. *Back Lett* 1999;14:109–115.
58. Marras WS. *Toward an understanding of dynamic variables in ergonomics. Occupational med: state of the arts review.* 1992;7:655–677.

59. Solomonow M, Zhou B-H, Baratta RV, et al. Biomechanics of increased exposure to lumbar injury caused by cyclic loading. Part 1: Loss of reflexive muscular stabilization. *Spine* 1999;24:2426–2434.

60. Gedalia U, Solomonow M, Zhou B-H, et al. Biomechanics of increased exposure to lumbar injury caused by cyclic loading. Part 2: Recovery of reflexive muscular stability with rest. *Spine* 1999;24:2461–2467.

61. Hadler NM, Carey TS. Back belts in the workplace. *JAMA* 2000;284:2780–2781.

62. Wassell JT, et al. A prospective study of back belts for prevention of back pain and injury, *JAMA* 2000;284:2727–2732.

63. Vlacyen JWS, Kole-Sinjders AMJ, Rotteveel AM, et al. The role of fear of movement/(re) injury in pain disability. *J Occup Rehabil* 1995;5:235–252.

64. Fordyce WE. *Behavioral methods for chronic pain and illness.* St. Louis: CV Mosby, 1976.

65. Fordyce WE, Shelton JL, Dundore DE. The modification of avoidance learning in pain behaviors. *J Behav Med* 1982;5:405–414.

66. Waddell G. A new clinical model for the treatment of low back pain *Spine* 1987;12:632–644.

67. Turk DC, Meichenbaum D, Genest M. *Pain and behavior medicine: a cognitive-behavior perspective.* New York: Guilford Press, 1983.

68. Nachemson AL. Newest knowledge of low back pain. *Clin Orthop* 1992;2:8–20.

69. Bortz WM. The disuse syndrome. *West J Med* 1984;141:691–694.

70. Wall PD. On the relationship of injury to pain. *Pain* 1979;6:253–264.

71. Flor H, Birbaumer N, Turk DC. The psychobiology of chronic pain. *Adv Behav Res Ther* 1990:121:47–84.

72. Romano JM, Turner JA. Chronic pain and depression: does the evidence support a relationship? *Psychol Bull* 1985;97:18–34.

73. Feuerstein M. A multidiscipline approach to the prevention, evaluation and management of work disability. *J Occup Rehabil* 1991;1:5–12.

74. Pilowsli I. Pain and illness behavior: assessment and management. In: Wall PD, Melzack R eds. *Textbook of pain.* Edinburgh: Churchill Livingstone, 1994.

75. Lethem J, Slade PD, Troup JDG, et al. Outline of a fear-avoidance model of exaggerated pain perception. *Behav Res Ther* 1983;21:401–408.

76. Kori SH, Miller RP, Todd DD. "Kinesiophobia": a new view of chronic pain behavior. *Pain Manage* 1990; 35–43.

77. Vlaeyen JWS, Geurts SM, Kole-Snijders AMJ. What do chronic pain patients think of their pain? Towards a pain cognition questionnaire. *Br J Clin Psychol* 1990;29:383–394.

78. Moon S, Liu J. The physician/patient encounter from a cognitive behavioral therapy perspective. *J Occup Rehabil* 1998;8:153–172.

79. Ashworth C, Williamson P, Montano D. A scale to measure physicians beliefs about psychosocial aspects of patient care. *Soc Sci Med* 1984;19:1235–1238.

80. Allman RM, Yoel WC, Clair JM. Reconciling the agendas of physicians and patients. In: Clair JM, Allman RM, eds. *Sociomedical perspectives on patient care.* Lexington, KY: The University Press of Kentucky, 1993:29–46.

81. Waitzkin H. Doctor-patient communication: clinical implications of social scientific research. *JAMA* 1984;252:2441–2446.

82. Kaplan S, Greenfield S, Ware J. Assessing the effects of physician-patient interactions on outcomes of chronic disease. *Med Care* 1989; S110–S127.
83. Roter DL, Hall JA, Katz NR. Relations between physician's behavior and patient's satisfaction, recall and impressions. *Med Care* 1987;25:437–451.
84. Dobson KS. *Handbook of cognitive-behavioral therapies.* New York: Guilford Press, 1988.
85. Waddell G, Main CJ, Morris EW, et al. Chronic low back pain. *Spine* 1987;12:632–644.
86. The Undesirable Patient. Editorial, *J Chronic Dis* 1970;22:777–779.
87. Vlaeyen JWS, Linton SJ. Fear-avoidance and its consequences in chronic musculoskeletal pain: the state of the art. Review article. *Pain* 2000;85:317–332.
88. Working off low back pain. *Lancet* 2000;355:1929–1930.
89. Von Korff M, Moore JC. Stepped care for back pain: activating approaches for primary care. *Ann Intern Med* 2001;134:911–917.
90. Muggleton JM, Kondracki M, Allen R. Spinal fusion for lumbar instability: does it have a scientific basis? *J Spinal Disord* 2000;13:3: 200–204.
91. Biering-Sorensen F, Bendix AF. Working off low back pain. *Lancet* 2000;355:1929–1930.
92. Von Korff M, Moore JC. Stepped care for low back pain: activating approaches for primary care. *Ann Intern Med* 2001;9:911–917.
93. Ahn S-H, Cho Y-W, Ahn M-W, et al. mRNA expression of cytokines and chemokines in herniated lumbar intervertebral discs. *Spine* 2002; 27:911–917.
94. Hashizume H, DeLeo JA, Colburn RW, Weinstein JN. Spinal glial activation and cytokine expression after lumbar root injury in the rat. *Spine* 2000;25:1206–1217.
95. Adamopoulos S, Parissis J, Karatzas D, et al. Physical training modulates proinflammatory cytokines and the soluble Fas/soluble Fas ligand system in patients with chronic heart failure. *J Am Coll Cardiol* 2002;39:653–663.
96. DeLeo JA, Yezierski RP. The role of neuroinflammation and neuro-immune activation in persistent pain. *Pain* 2001;90:1–6.
97. Kawaguchi S, Yamashita T, Katahira G, et al. Chemokine profile of herniated intervertebral discs infiltrated with monocytes and macrophages. *Spine* 2002;15;27:1511–1516.
98. Kawaguchi S, Yamashita T, Yokogushi K, et al. Immunophenotypic analysis of the inflammatory infiltrates in herniated intervertebral discs. *Spine* 2001;26:1209–1214.
99. Hashizume H, DeLeo JA, Colburn RW, et al. Spinal glial activation and cytokine expression after lumbar root injury in the rat. *Spine* 2000; 25:1206–1217.
100. Arruda JL, Colburn RW, Rickman AJ, et al. Increase of interleukin-6 mRNA in the spinal cord following peripheral nerve injury in the rat: potential role of IL-6 in neuropathic pain. *Mol Brain Res* 1998;62:228–235.
101. Holers VM. Complement. In: Rich RR, Fleisher TA, Schwartz, et al., eds. *Clinical immunology: principles and practice.* St Louis: Mosby-Year Book, 1996.
102. DeLeo JA, Colburn RW, Nichols M, et al. Interleukin-6-mediated hyperalgesia/allodynia and increased spinal IL-6 expression in a rat mononeuropathy model. *J Interferon Cytokine Res* 1996;16:695–700.

103. Kiefer R, Lindholm D, Kreutzberg GW. Interleukin-6 and transforming growth factor-beta 1 mRNAs are induced in rat facial nucleus following motoneuron axotomy. *Eur J Neurosci* 1993;5:775–781.
104. Hariri RJ, Chang VA, Barie PS, et al. Traumatic injury induces interleukin-6 production by human astrocytes. *Brain Res* 1994;636:139–142.
105. Shohami E, Novikov M, Bass R, et al. Closed head injury triggers early production of TNF alpha and IL-6 by brain tissue. *J Cereb Blood Flow Metab* 1994;14:615–619.
106. Woodroofe MN, Sarna GS, Wadhwa M, et al. Detection of interleukin-1 and interleukin-6 in adult rat brain, following mechanical injury, by in vivo microdialysis: evidence of a role for microglia in cytokine production. *J Neuroimmunol* 1991;33:227–236.
107. DeLeo JA, Colburn RW, Nichols M, et al. Interleukin-6-mediated hyperalgesia/allodynia and increased spinal IL-6 expression in a rat mononeuropathy model. *J Interferon Cytokine Res* 1996;16:695–700.
108. Winkelstein BA, Rutkowski MD, Weinstein JN, et al. Quantification of neural tissue injury in a rat radiculopathy model: comparison of local deformation, behavioral outcomes, and spinal cytokine mRNA for two surgeons. *J Neurosci Methods* 2001;111:49–57.
109. Korhonen T, et al. Treatment of sciatica with infliximab, a monoclonal chimaeric antibody against TNF-alpha, presented at the annual meeting of the International Society for the Study of the Lumbar Spine, Cleveland 2002: as yet unpublished.
110. Will a new treatment revolutionize the treatment of sciatica: and Preventing nerve root damage with TNF-alpha inhibitors- two studies in animals. *Back Lett* 2001;16:121, 128–130.
111. The BACK letter. Biological treatment for sciatica produces dramatic results in a human pilot study. *Back Lett* 2002;17:7:73–81.
112. Kawaguchi S, Yamashita T, Katahira GK, et al. Chemokine profile of herniated intervertebral discs infiltrated with monocytes and macrophages. *Spine* 2002;27:1511–1516.
113. Haro H, Shinomiya K, Komori H, et al. Upregulated expression of chemokines in herniated nucleus pulposus resorption. *Spine* 1996; 21:1647–52.
114. Kikuchi T, Nakamura T, Ikeda T, et al. Monocyte chemoattractant protein-1 in the intervertebral disc. *Spine* 1998;23:1091–1099.

SUBJECT INDEX

Page numbers followed by *f* denote figures. Page numbers followed by *t* denote tables.

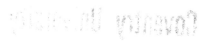